```
||||||||||||||||||||||||||||||||||||||||||||||||||||
MW00562443
```

ITI Treatment Guide
Volume 7

ITI
Treatment
Guide

Editors:
S. Chen, D. Buser, D. Wismeijer

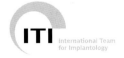
ITI International Team
for Implantology

Authors:
L. Cordaro, H. Terheyden

Volume 7

Ridge Augmentation Procedures in Implant Patients
A Staged Approach

Quintessence Publishing Co, Ltd
Berlin, Chicago, London, Tokyo, Barcelona, Beijing,
Istanbul, Milan, Moscow, New Delhi, Paris, Prague,
São Paulo, Seoul, Singapore, Warsaw

German National Library CIP Data

The German National Library has listed this publication in the German National Bibliography. Detailed bibliographical data are available at http://dnb.ddb.de.

© 2014 Quintessence Publishing Co, Ltd
Ifenpfad 2 – 4, 12107 Berlin, Germany
www.quintessenz.de

Illustrations: Ute Drewes, CH-Basel,
                    www.drewes.ch
Copyediting: Triacom Dental, D-Barendorf,
                    www.dental.triacom.com
Graphic Concept: Wirz Corporate AG, CH-Zürich
Production: Juliane Richter, D-Berlin
Printing: Bosch-Druck GmbH, D-Landshut,
                    www.bosch-druck.de

Printed in Germany
ISBN: 978-3-86867-217-6

The materials offered in the ITI Treatment Guide are for educational purposes only and intended as a step-by-step guide to treatment of a particular case and patient situation. These recommendations are based on conclusions of the ITI Consensus Conferences and, as such, in line with the ITI treatment philosophy. These recommendations, nevertheless, represent the opinions of the authors. Neither the ITI nor the authors, editors and publishers make any representation or warranty for the completeness or accuracy of the published materials and as a consequence do not accept any liability for damages (including, without limitation, direct, indirect, special, consequential or incidental damages or loss of profits) caused by the use of the information contained in the ITI Treatment Guide. The information contained in the ITI Treatment Guide cannot replace an individual assessment by a clinician, and its use for the treatment of patients is therefore in the sole responsibility of the clinician.

The inclusion of or reference to a particular product, method, technique or material relating to such products, methods, or techniques in the ITI Treatment Guide does not represent a recommendation or an endorsement of the values, features, or claims made by its respective manufacturers.

Some of the manufacturer and product names referred to in this publication may be registered trademarks or proprietary names, even though specific reference to this fact is not made. Therefore, the appearance of a name without designation as proprietary is not to be construed as a representation by the publisher that it is in the public domain.

The tooth identification system used in this ITI Treatment Guide is that of the FDI World Dental Federation.

The ITI Mission is ...

"... to promote and disseminate knowledge on all aspects of implant dentistry and related tissue regeneration through education and research to the benefit of the patient."

Preface

A fundamental requirement for successful treatment outcomes with dental implants is the presence of an adequate bone volume to support the required number and distribution of osseointegrated implants. When bone volume is deficient due to ridge atrophy, trauma, or pathoses, implant therapy may not be possible unless the alveolar ridge is augmented sufficiently.

The present Volume 7 of the ITI Treatment Guide series has been compiled to provide clinicians with the latest evidence-based information on techniques and materials utilized for ridge augmentation at healed sites.

An up-to-date analysis of the current evidence is based in part on the proceedings of the 4th ITI Consensus Conference in Stuttgart in 2008, and a review of the current literature. A detailed discussion on preoperative assessment is presented, followed by an in-depth description of the methods and materials used for ridge augmentation.

Twelve clinical cases—presented by clinicians from around the world—demonstrate the planning and treatment principles for successfully rehabilitating patients with varying degrees of ridge atrophy.

Volume 7 of the ITI Treatment Guide series continues the tradition and mission of the ITI "... to promote and disseminate knowledge on all aspects of implant dentistry to the benefit of the patient."

S. Chen   D. Buser   D. Wismeijer

Acknowledgment

We would like to thank Mr. Thomas Kiss of the ITI Center for his invaluable assistance in the preparation of this volume of the Treatment Guide series. We would also like to express our gratitude to Ms. Juliane Richter (Quintessence Publishing) for typesetting and for coordinating the production workflow, Mr. Per N. Döhler (Triacom Dental) for their editing support, and Ms. Ute Drewes for her excellent illustrations. We also acknowledge continuing support from Straumann AG, ITI's corporate partner.

Editors and Authors

Editors:

Stephen Chen
  MDSc, PhD
  School of Dental Science
  University of Melbourne
  720 Swanston Street
  Melbourne, VIC 3010, Australia
  E-mail: schen@balwynperio.com.au

Daniel Buser
  DDS, Prof Dr med dent
  Chair, Department of Oral Surgery and Stomatology
  University of Bern School of Dental Medicine
  Freiburgstrasse 7
  3010 Bern, Switzerland
  E-mail: daniel.buser@zmk.unibe.ch

Daniel Wismeijer
  DDS, PhD, Professor
  Head, Section of Implantology and
  Prosthetic Dentistry
  Department of Oral Function and
  Restorative Dentistry
  Academic Centre for Dentistry Amsterdam (ACTA)
  Free University
  Louwesweg 1
  1066 EA Amsterdam, Netherlands
  E-mail: d.wismeijer@acta.nl

Authors:

Luca Cordaro
  MD, DDS, PhD
  Head, Department of Periodontics and
  Prosthodontics
  Eastman Dental Hospital Roma and Studio Cordaro
  Via Guido d'Arezzo 2
  00198 Roma, Italy
  E-mail: lucacordaro@usa.net

Hendrik Terheyden
  MD, DDS, Dr med, Dr med dent, Professor
  Department of Oral and Maxillofacial Surgery
  Red Cross Hospital
  Hansteinstrasse 29
  34121 Kassel, Germany
  E-mail: terheyden@rkh-kassel.de

Contributors

Daniel Buser
DDS, Prof Dr med dent
Chair, Department of Oral Surgery and Stomatology
University of Bern School of Dental Medicine
Freiburgstrasse 7
3010 Bern, Switzerland
E-mail: daniel.buser@zmk.unibe.ch

Urs C. Belser
DMD, Prof Dr med dent
Chairman emeritus
Department of Prosthodontics
University of Geneva School of Dental Medicine
Rue Barthelémy-Menn 19
1205 Geneva, Switzerland
E-mail: urs.belser@unige.ch

Emma L Lewis
BDS, MBBS
55 Labouchere Road
South Perth, WA 6151, Australia
E-mail: ellewis67@gmail.com

Frank Lozano
DMD, MS
2441 NW 43rd Street Suite 16
Gainesville, FL 32606, USA
E-mail: champuf@aol.com

Paolo Casentini
DDS, Dr med dent
Narcodont
Piazza S. Ambrogio 16
20123 Milano, Italy
E-mail: paolocasentini@fastwebnet.it

Bruno Schmid
Dr med dent
Bayweg 3
3123 Belp, Switzerland
E-mail: brunoschmid@vtxmail.ch

Waldemar D. Polido
DDS, MS, PhD
Oral and Maxillofacial Surgery/Implant Dentistry
Hospital Moinhos de Vento and
Contento – Odontologia Especializada
R. Marcelo Gama, 1148
Porto Alegre, RS, Brazil
E-mail: cirurgia.implantes@polido.com.br

Paulo Eduardo Pittas do Canto
DDS
Prosthodontics
Contento – Odontologia Especializada
R. Marcelo Gama, 1148
Porto Alegre, RS, Brazil
E-Mail: pittasdocanto@terra.com.br

Mario Roccuzzo
   DMD, Dr med dent
   Corso Tassoni 14
   10143 Torino, Italy
   E-mail: mroccuzzo@iol.it

Luca Cordaro
   MD, DDS, PhD
   Head, Department of Periodontics and
   Prosthodontics
   Eastman Dental Hospital Roma and Studio Cordaro
   Via Guido d'Arezzo 2
   00198 Roma, Italy
   E-mail: lucacordaro@usa.net

Dieter Weingart
   Dr med, Dr med dent, Professor
   Department of Maxillofacial Surgery
   Klinikum Stuttgart, Katharinenhospital
   Kriegsbergstraße 60
   70174 Stuttgart, Germany
   E-mail: d.weingart@klinikum-stuttgart.de

Yong-Dae Kwon
   DMD, MSD, PhD, Professor
   Department of Oral and Maxillofacial Surgery
   Kyung Hee University School of Dentistry
   26 Kyungheedae-ro, Dongdaemun-gu
   130-701 Seoul, Korea
   E-mail: yongdae.kwon@gmail.com

Matteo Chiapasco
   MD, Professor
   Head, Unit of Oral Surgery
   School of Dentistry and Stomatology
   San Paolo Hospital, University of Milan
   Via Beldiletto 1/3
   20142 Milano, Italy
   E-mail: matteo.chiapasco@unimi.it

João Emílio Roehe Neto
   DDS
   Rua Soledade, 569/1110, Torre Beta
   Porto Alegre, RS, Brazil
   E-mail: jemiliorn@gmail.com

Hendrik Terheyden
   MD, DDS, Dr med, Dr med dent, Professor
   Department of Oral and Maxillofacial Surgery
   Red Cross Hospital
   Hansteinstrasse 29
   34121 Kassel, Germany
   E-mail: terheyden@rkh-kassel.de

Table of Contents

1 Introduction

H. Terheyden, L. Cordaro

Augmentation procedures to increase the volume of deficient or atrophic alveolar bone have been extensively described in the literature. They are widely performed by numerous surgeons all over the world in an effort to safely place implants where they can support an adequate functional and esthetic prosthesis.

The past few years have seen the development of surgical techniques to deal with bone defects of almost any shape or size, regardless of whether they result from ridge atrophy, trauma, inflammation, tumors, or malformation. Ridge augmentation may, however, run up against limitations and complications for a number of reasons, such as general health issues, dental status, extent and location of the bone defect, patient preference, reluctance to undergo major surgical procedures, or budget considerations.

Generally speaking, the prognoses for implant survival are no less favorable in regenerated bone than in pristine bone.

Ridge augmentation serves three primary objectives:

- Function: to create a volume of vital bone that will accommodate a dental implant sufficiently long and wide for its ideal restorative and functional position.
- Esthetics: to give the associated soft tissues the bony support needed for an esthetic appearance of gingival/mucosal and facial structures.
- Prognosis: to create sufficient bone volume coronally around the neck of the implant to cover the endosseous implant segment, ensuring a tight soft-tissue seal and a predictable long-term prognosis of the implant.

Secondary goals in selecting a specific approach would be to keep the surgical technique straightforward, to minimize the surgical and postoperative burden for the patient, to ensure low morbidity, and to reduce the number of surgical sessions. Consideration is also given to cost, predictability, and healing time. Clinicians should realize that there may be one or several restorative options to meet the functional and esthetic requirements of a given patient. It is the treatment provider's responsibility to study these options, propose the best solution and then present the patient with the expected outcome of this favored restorative strategy either in the form of a provisional denture setup and try-in or within an appropriate software environment. In doing so, the patient will have a clear understanding and no misconceptions about the appearance of the final prosthesis. This early preview of the treatment endpoint will clearly disclose any need for bone augmentation procedures to correct deficiencies in the underlying hard and soft tissues.

Anticipating patient requirements in this way has come to be known as "backward planning" and the treatment strategies derived from it as "restoration-driven" (or "prosthetically driven") approaches. It is part of this rationale that a dentist, rather than accepting a restorative compromise, should consider reconstructing the bone to meet the restorative needs.

Also, there should be no reason for clinicians to withhold from their patients useful procedures of bone augmentation merely because they personally lack the skills to conduct these procedures on their own. It is better to refer a patient to an oral or maxillofacial surgeon than to accept a compromise that may be limiting to the restorative outcome. That said, the referring clinician should still have a good knowledge in the basics of bone augmentation and related options to advise their patients correctly, and it is important to ensure good collaboration between all members of the clinical team.

The focus of this volume will be on procedures of ridge augmentation performed on healed sites in preparation for delayed implant placement. This approach, here called the "staged" approach (which does not imply that the augmentation procedure itself consists of multiple stages) differs from simultaneous procedures of bone augmentation and implant placement in that they are broken down into an initial surgical session to augment the ridge and a second session for implant placement further down the line. The simultaneous approach is not extensively discussed in this volume. Procedures of sinus floor elevation have been covered extensively in Volume 6 of this ITI Treatment Guide series, and the reader is referred to Volume 3 for details on bone augmentation to support implant procedures in post-extraction sites.

It is the authors' ambition to provide the reader with a systematic way of assessing bone defects that may underlie specific clinical situations and to offer guidelines toward selecting the most appropriate surgical strategies to deal with specific defect types.

2 Consensus Statements on Ridge Augmentation and Review of the Literature

Various groups were appointed to deal with different topics at the 4th ITI Consensus Conference in Stuttgart in 2008. Group 4 was assigned to review surgical techniques and biomaterials used in implant dentistry and to evaluate the available evidence supporting their use. Two of four review papers that had been prepared for Group 4 were devoted to materials and methods for ridge augmentation:

- Simon Storgård Jensen and Hendrik Terheyden: *Bone augmentation procedures in localized defects in the alveolar ridge: Clinical results with different bone grafts and bone-substitute materials. A review* (Jensen and Terheyden 2009)
- Matteo Chiapasco, Paolo Casentini and Marco Zaniboni: *Bone augmentation procedures in implant dentistry* (Chiapasco and coworkers 2009).

These review papers formed the basis for discussing and subsequently formulating a series of consensus statements and recommendations for clinical procedures (Chen and coworkers 2009). Section 2.1 summarizes the consensus statements and clinical recommendations pertaining to ridge augmentation procedures. Section 2.2 will then update the reader on the more recent literature that has been added since these consensus statements were published in 2009.

2.1 Consensus Statements and Treatment Guidelines Formulated at the 2008 ITI Consensus Conference

2.1.1 Consensus Statements

General statements

- Several surgical procedures are available and effective for the augmentation of deficient edentulous ridges to allow implants to be placed. However, most of the studies are retrospective in nature, with small sample sizes and short follow-up periods.
- Therefore, direct comparisons between studies should not be made and definitive conclusions cannot be drawn.
- There are a variety of defect situations with increasing complexity ranging from fenestrations, to dehiscences, to lateral deficiencies, and to vertical deficiencies including combinations of these.
- There are a variety of augmentation materials available with different biologic and mechanical properties ranging from particulate alloplastic materials to intraorally harvested block grafts.
- Survival rates of implants placed in regenerated bone after treatment of localized defects in the alveolar ridge are comparable to survival rates of implants placed in native bone.
- It was not possible to demonstrate the superiority of one augmentation technique over another based on implant survival rates.

Dehiscence- and fenestration-type defects

- Augmentation of dehiscence- and fenestration-type defects is effective in reducing the amount of exposed implant surface. Complete resolution of dehiscence and fenestrationtype defects cannot be predictably accomplished irrespective of the grafting protocol employed.
- Increased defect fill was observed when the augmentation procedure included the use of a barrier membrane.
- Survival rates of implants placed simultaneously with augmentation of dehiscence or fenestration type defects are high.

Horizontal ridge augmentation

- Techniques are available to effectively and predictably increase the width of the alveolar ridge.
- Augmentation utilizing autologous bone blocks with or without membranes results in higher gains in ridge width and lower complication rates than the use of particulate materials with or without a membrane.
- Survival rates of implants placed in horizontally augmented alveolar ridges are high.

Vertical ridge augmentation

- Techniques are available to increase the height of the alveolar ridge. However, their predictability is substantially lower compared to horizontal ridge augmentation procedures.
- Augmentation utilizing autologous bone blocks with or without membranes results in higher gains in ridge height than the use of particulate materials with or without a membrane.
- The complication rate related to vertical augmentation of the alveolar ridge is substantially higher compared to horizontal ridge augmentation procedures.
- Survival rates of implants placed in vertically augmented alveolar ridges are high.

Maxillary sinus floor elevation using the transalveolar approach

- Maxillary sinus floor elevation using the transalveolar approach is predictable for augmenting bone in the posterior maxilla.
- A variety of grafting materials can be safely and predictably used, alone or in combination. These materials include autografts, allografts, xenografts, and alloplastic materials.
- At present, it is not clear whether the introduction of a grafting material improves the prognosis.

Onlay bone grafting of extended resorption of edentulous ridges

- Autologous onlay bone grafting procedures are effective and predictable for the correction of severely resorbed edentulous ridges to allow implant placement. An uneventful healing/consolidation of grafts taken from intra- and/or extraoral donor sites occurs in the majority of cases.
- Acceptable survival rates of implants placed in maxillae and mandibles reconstructed with autologous onlay bone grafts are reported. The survival rates are slightly lower than those of implants placed in native bone.

Maxillary sinus floor elevation using the lateral approach

- Maxillary sinus floor elevation procedures are predictable for augmenting bone in the posterior maxilla.
- A variety of grafting materials can be safely and predictably used, alone or in combination. These materials include autografts, allografts, xenografts, and alloplastic materials.
- The use of autografts does not influence survival rates of rough surface implants, but may reduce healing times.
- The quantity and quality of bone in the residual maxilla influence survival rates of implants independently from the type of grafting procedure.
- Survival rates of rough surface implants placed in augmented maxillary sinuses are similar to those of implants inserted in native bone.

Split-ridge/ridge expansion techniques with simultaneous implant placement

- Split-ridge and expansion techniques are effective for the correction of moderately resorbed edentulous ridges in selected cases.
- Survival rates of implants placed at sites augmented using split-ridge/ridge expansion techniques are similar to those of implants inserted in native bone.

Split-ridge technique with interpositional bone grafts

- There is a lack of evidence concerning the split-ridge technique with interpositional bone graft and delayed implant placement.

Vertical distraction osteogenesis

- Alveolar distraction osteogenesis can be used to augment vertically deficient alveolar ridges in selected cases.
- Alveolar distraction osteogenesis has a high rate of complications. These include change of the distracting vector, incomplete distraction, fracture of the distracting device, and partial relapse of the initial bone gain.

- Survival rates of implants placed at sites augmented using distraction osteogenesis are similar to those of implants inserted in native bone.

Le Fort I osteotomy with interpositional autologous bone grafts

- Le Fort I osteotomy with interpositional autologous bone graft can be used successfully to treat atrophy of the maxilla including cases associated with severe intermaxillary discrepancy.

2.1.2 Treatment Guidelines

- Bone augmentation procedures should always follow a prosthetically driven plan to allow ideal three-dimensional implant positioning. The concept of "prosthetically driven bone augmentation" should be taken into consideration whenever possible.

Localized defects

- Dehiscence and fenestration-type defects may be successfully managed using a particulate autograft or bone substitute covered with a membrane.
- Horizontal ridge augmentations often require the use of an autologous block graft, which may be combined with a membrane and/or a particulate autograft or bone substitute.
- Vertical ridge augmentations most often require the use of an autologous block graft, which may be combined with a membrane and/or a particulate autograft, allograft, or xenograft. Despite the use of an autologous block graft, elevated rates of complications, including graft resorption, and a need for additional grafting have to be anticipated. Even localized vertical bone deficiencies may require advanced surgical procedures like distraction osteogenesis, interpositional grafts, or onlay grafts from extraoral donor sites.
- The clinician should be aware that the obtainable defect fill decreases and complication rates and need for additional grafting procedures increase with more demanding defect types. The augmentation material should be selected according to the biological and mechanical characteristics needed in the specific clinical situation.
- The use of a membrane is indicated whenever a particulate material is applied.

Autologous onlay bone grafting of severely resorbed edentulous ridges

- Onlay bone grafting is a technique-sensitive procedure and is recommended only for well-trained clinicians.
- Both intraoral donor sites (including the mental symphysis, the mandibular body and ramus, and the

maxillary tuberosity) and extraoral donor sites (including the iliac crest and the calvarium) can be used for collecting autologous bone.

- The choice between intraoral and extraoral sites is mainly related to the quantity of bone necessary to reconstruct the deficient alveolar ridge. Preference should be given to donor sites where the cortical component is more prevalent, in order to reduce the risk of early or late resorption of the graft.
- Bone harvesting from the mental symphysis is associated with relevant morbidity, and the quantity of available bone is frequently limited. Neural damage to the incisal nerve occurs frequently. Therefore, the mental symphysis should not be the first choice for harvesting.
- Bone harvesting from the maxillary tuberosity is followed by low morbidity but is not well documented. The quality and quantity of available bone is often poor. Indications are limited to reconstruction of small defects.
- Bone harvesting from the mandibular ramus offers good quality and quantity of available bone, due to the possibility of harvesting from both sides.
- Bone harvesting from the iliac crest offers high quantities of bone. However, the cancellous bone component is dominant and may be associated with a higher risk of unpredictable bone resorption. When bone is harvested from the anterior iliac crest there may be associated transient gait disturbances.
- Bone harvesting from the calvarium offers greater quantities of highly corticalized bone and is associated with low morbidity.
- Accurate modeling and stabilization of the graft with screws, and tension-free primary closure of the overlying flaps, are fundamental to the success of the procedure. Overcorrection of the defect is recommended to compensate for the potential risk of bone resorption. Coverage of the bone grafts with a low-resorption-rate xenograft/alloplastic material, with or without a membrane, may be indicated to reduce bone resorption.
- The economic and biologic costs of bone transplantation must be carefully weighed. In selected clinical situations short and/or reduced-diameter implants may be considered instead.
- The severely atrophic edentulous maxilla frequently needs bone grafts due to poor quality of the residual bone and the presence of pneumatized cavities, including the maxillary sinus and the nose.
- Both implant placement in conjunction with bone grafting and delayed implant placement have been proposed. Delayed implant placement is recommended.

Split-ridge/ridge-expansion techniques

- Split-ridge/ridge-expansion techniques are indicated in selected situations where atrophy of the edentulous ridge has developed horizontally and cancellous bone is present between the oral and facial cortical plates, and adequate residual height exists.
- Excessive facial inclination of the alveolar ridge may contraindicate this procedure, as it may worsen the initial situation from a prosthetic point of view.
- The presence of undercuts may increase the risk of bone fracture.
- This technique is mainly indicated in the maxilla. Ridge expansion in the mandible is frequently difficult due to the brittleness of the bone.

Vertical distraction osteogenesis

- Vertical distraction osteogenesis is a technique-sensitive procedure and is recommended for well-trained clinicians.
- Indications of this technique should be limited to vertically deficient ridges with adequate residual width. As the segment to be distracted has to be at least 3 mm in height, severely deficient mandibles are not good candidates due to the risk of neural damage and/or mandibular fracture.
- The presence of maxillary sinus and/or nasal cavities may be contraindications.
- The rigidity of the palatal mucosa may negatively influence the distraction vector.

Le Fort I osteotomy with interpositional autologous bone grafts

- Le Fort I osteotomy with interpositional autologous bone grafts is indicated in cases of extremely severe resorption, and where there is an unfavorable horizontal and vertical intermaxillary relationship.
- This procedure is technique-sensitive and is recommended for well-trained clinicians.

Sinus floor elevation using the lateral approach

- In sites with limited initial bone height not allowing insertion of the desired implant length, sinus floor elevation via the lateral approach can be used to increase the bone height.
- As atrophy of the maxilla occurs three-dimensionally, the edentulous posterior maxilla should not only be evaluated in terms of initial bone height below the maxillary sinus but also in relation to any vertical and horizontal ridge deficiencies. If relevant vertical/horizontal intermaxillary discrepancy is present, an onlay bone augmentation may be considered to create both sufficient bone volume and proper intermaxillary relationships, to optimize implant placement and related prosthetic restoration.

- Data related to the initial clinical situation should be reported, and defects classified according to well-defined criteria.
- If the initial bone height allows primary implant stability, simultaneous implant placement (one surgical stage) can be recommended. In situations where primary stability cannot be achieved, the elevation of the sinus floor should be performed in a separate surgical procedure followed by delayed implant insertion (two surgical stages).
- Rough-surfaced implants should be utilized. Coverage of the access window with a membrane may be considered when bone substitutes are used as the only grafting material.

Sinus floor elevation using the transalveolar approach
- Sinus floor elevation using the transalveolar approach can be recommended in sites with sufficient alveolar crest width, initial bone height of 5 mm or more, and relatively flat sinus floor anatomy.
- The main disadvantage of this technique is possible perforation of the sinus membrane, which is difficult to detect and to manage. Therefore, the transalveolar technique should only be performed by clinicians with experience in performing sinus floor elevation via the lateral approach.
- A prerequisite for using this technique is that primary implant stability is achieved.

2.1.3 Treatment Outcomes

The following treatment outcomes were reported for the 4th ITI Consensus Conference in the review papers of Jensen and Terheyden (2009) and Chiapasco and coworkers (2009).

Treatment of dehiscence defects
Clinical treatments of dehiscence defects were associated with 5-year implant survival rates of 94% to 100% depending on the methods applied. Defect fill varied between 76% and 79% when a barrier membrane was used without filler. In the presence of a filler, defect fill varied between 84% and 87%, the best results being obtained with deproteinized bovine bone mineral (DBBM) in the form of Bio-Oss® (Geistlich, Waldenburg, Switzerland) in conjunction with a resorbable non-crosslinked collagen membrane (Bio-Gide®; Geistlich).

Staged horizontal ridge augmentation
Staged procedures of horizontal ridge augmentation were associated with 5-year implant survival rates of 97% to 100% depending on the methods applied. Gains in ridge width varied between 3.2 and 4.7 mm depending on the materials used. The best results were obtained with mixtures of DBBM and particulated autologous bone, including the use of a resorbable membrane. The smallest gains in width were reported with allografts.

Staged vertical ridge augmentation
Staged procedures of vertical ridge augmentation were associated with 5-year implant survival rates of 97% to 100% depending on the methods applied. Gains in ridge height varied between 3.6 and 9.2 mm depending on the materials used. The greatest gains were obtained with iliac onlay grafts and the smallest ones with mixtures of DBBM and particulated autologous bone.

Complication rates
Complication rates of 12% to 26% were reported for single-stage augmentation of dehiscence defects, mainly including soft-tissue dehiscences and wound infections. The highest rates of membrane exposure were generally observed with membranes consisting of expanded polytetrafluoroethylene (ePTFE).

Staged procedures of horizontal augmentation were found to involve a wide variety of complication rates, averaging between 5% and 43% across the reviewed studies. The 43% rate was again reported for ePTFE membranes and was mainly a function of membrane exposure. For the other materials, the mean complication rates were generally 5%.

Vertical procedures involved higher complication rates than horizontal ones, ranging from 14 to 26% of cases. The lowest rate was identified for intraoral block grafts, the highest rate for iliac bone harvesting – the latter predominantly involving complications of postoperative pain at the donor site and gait disturbances.

2.2 Literature Review

L. Cordaro

Several reviews have been devoted to alveolar bone augmentation techniques. Most of the studies were intended to demonstrate the usefulness of specific techniques of alveolar bone reconstruction by reporting treatment outcomes, complications, and success rates for the reconstructed bone areas, the inserted implants, and perhaps the prostheses (Jensen and Terheyden 2009; Chiapasco and coworkers 2009; Aghaloo and Moy 2007).

The results of these systematic reviews indicate that numerous reconstructive techniques have been demonstrated to be relatively safe and effective, including:

- Grafting with autologous bone blocks
- Lateral sinus floor elevation with bone grafting materials
- Transcrestal sinus floor elevation with osteotomes or other purpose-designed instruments
- Simultaneous or staged GBR with barrier membranes and bone grafts and/or substitutes
- Horizontal ridge splitting/expansion with osteotomes or devices
- Vertical or horizontal distraction osteogenesis
- Osteotomies with jaw repositioning and grafting

Staged or simultaneous procedures to augment the jawbone are widely performed with different techniques and varying outcomes by clinicians around the world.

However, since the majority of these clinical studies were not governed by well-defined inclusion criteria, most of the available data have to do with the augmentation procedures themselves without focusing on the clinical baseline situations. Some studies on GBR, for instance, reported treatment outcomes in patients with partially and completely edentulous jaws who had presented with dissimilar defect types at baseline. This lack of information on initial defect situations makes it difficult for clinicians to arrive at evidence-based decisions about what

method of augmentation they should preferably use on a given clinical defect.

This volume of the Treatment Guide series is intended to guide clinicians faced with different types of edentulism and defect types in selecting the most appropriate clinical procedure in each clinical situation. In Chapter 3, a classification of the defect-types will be presented, and in Chapter 4 a schematic description of the preferred surgical approach for the given baseline clinical situation will be provided. These clinical recommendations are based on the outcomes of a recent systematic review which was undertaken to identify the clinical indications for various bone augmentation procedures in relation to defect type and dimensions (Milincovic and Cordaro 2013).

The literature search for this review was performed in the Medline (PubMed) and Cochrane Library databases, using search criteria that returned any pertinent clinical trials published between 1990 and 2012, and supplemented by a hand search of the most relevant journals.

All types of clinical investigations were considered, including controlled clinical trials with or without randomization, prospective and retrospective studies and including papers that presented data on augmentation volumes while not reporting all outcome measures.

Inclusion criteria
- Information on defect type (fenestration defects, dehiscence defects, vertical or horizontal or combined defects in partially or completely edentulous jaws)
- Information on pre- and postoperative ridge dimensions and on bone gains

Applicable criteria for completely edentulous jaws were confined to information on ridge and defect characteristics and on bone gains.

Exclusion criteria

- Surgery performed simultaneously with immediate implant placement into fresh extraction sockets (type 1, ITI classification)
- Sinus floor augmentation without additional ridge augmentation
- Case reports
- Reports on techniques not disclosing clinical outcomes
- Studies providing histological data only
- Surgery preceded by peri-implantitis, trauma, tumor ablation, or treatment of various medical syndromes

Treatment outcomes extracted for review

- Pre- and postoperative defect sizes and/or postoperative bone gains (reported as defect fill or linear bone gain)
- Implant survival and success rates at augmented sites
- Implant failure rates
- Complication rates

All studies meeting the inclusion criteria were grouped by types of edentulism (partial or complete), defect types (fenestration, dehiscence, horizontal, vertical), and techniques of augmentation. In this way, the authors were able to relate the outcomes of augmentation procedures to defect types and dimensions. Studies not disclosing the initial situations were excluded because they offered no insights into indications for specific procedures.

2.2.1 Included Studies

The review included 35 studies on horizontal defects in partially edentulous cases—16 of them with GBR performed at the time of implant placement, 5 with staged GBR, 8 with block grafts, and 6 with ridge splitting/expansion. A total of 19 studies covered vertical defects in partially edentulous cases—4 with simultaneous GBR, 2 with staged GBR, 6 with block grafts, and 7 with distraction osteogenesis. Edentulous jaws were covered by 15 studies—9 with block grafting for vertical or horizontal augmentation or both, and 6 with Le Fort I osteotomies.

2.2.2 Patients with Partially Edentulous Jaws

By relating treatment outcomes reported for partially edentulous patients to initial clinical situations and augmentation techniques, some insights were gained into the performance of different approaches to specific defect types and dimensions. The main limitation affecting this part of the review was that not all papers contained detailed information to distinguish between single-tooth and extended edentulous spaces.

Fenestration and dehiscence defects

There is strong evidence supporting the use of GBR to handle a dehiscence or fenestration defect simultaneously with implant placement.

Horizontal defects

There is evidence supporting the use of staged GBR for horizontal augmentation in preparation for implant placement (after healing of the bone reconstruction) when the residual crest is at least 2.9 mm wide. Mean bone gain was 3.31 mm in the included studies, involving a 15% complication rate due to membrane exposure.

Scientific evidence is available to support the use of bone block grafts to augment horizontal defects in a staged approach when the ridge is 3.19 mm wide on average. This approach is documented to involve 4.3 mm of linear bone gain by the time of implant placement, with complication rates of 2.5% to 10% due to graft exposure.

The literature also provides evidence to support the use of ridge expansion/splitting techniques for horizontal augmentation of deficient ridges (mean ridge width: 3.37 mm). A mean linear bone gain of 2.95 mm is documented, involving a complication rate of 0.9% to 26% due to malfracture of the buccal bone plate.

Vertical defects

There is evidence that GBR performed at the time of implant placement yields effective augmentation when the initial circumferential vertical defect is 4.1 mm. A mean vertical bone gain of 3.04 mm has been achieved with this approach based on the included studies, with membrane exposure in 12.6% of cases.

Initial vertical defects of 4.7 mm will allow for a staged approach of GBR with delayed implant placement. A mean linear bone gain of 4.3 mm is documented after healing, including an 8% complication rate due to membrane exposure.

The use of bone block grafts is on record as yielding a mean linear bone gain of 4.7 mm, given a vertical augmentation requirement of at least 4 mm. A high complication rate should be anticipated, with graft exposure in 12.5% to 33.33% and complete loss of the graft in 8% to 20% of cases.

Evidence is also available for the use of distraction osteogenesis to correct vertical defects. Vertical bone gains of 7 mm have been achieved with this approach. The complication rate is relatively high, involving lingual inclination in 18% to 22%, persistent hypoesthesia in 2.9%, and additional need for grafting in 64.4% of cases.

Based on this systematic review, some specific clinical indications for the treatment of certain defect types in partially edentulous patients may be proposed.

Augmentation in horizontal defects. In horizontal defects with a crest wider than 4 mm and when only a dehiscence after implant placement is expected, simultaneous GBR (at the time of implant placement) is effective. When the crest is less than 3.5 mm, with a risk of placing the implant outside the bony envelope or with a reduced primary stability, a staged approach is mandatory and either GBR (with less augmentation potential) or bone blocks (that provide wider reconstructions but may need an additional harvesting procedure) may be successfully used. Ridge splitting or expansion can be used in the latter situation, but this technique is associated with a higher complication rate and a smaller amount of augmentation when compared to the previously mentioned techniques.

Augmentation in vertical defects. When treating vertical defects, the use of GBR simultaneously with implant placement is feasible when the initial vertical defect is up to 4 mm. For defects greater than 4 mm, a GBR procedure with non-simultaneous implant placement can be performed. Bone blocks have been used for treatment of vertical defects when at least 4 mm of vertical reconstruction was needed, with a possible mean vertical bone gain of 4.7 mm. It should be noted that although these vertical gains are achievable, the procedures are associated with elevated complication rates and require a high degree of clinical skill and experience to perform. Distraction osteogenesis is another treatment option for vertical alveolar ridge augmentation, where up to 7 mm vertical bone gain can be expected. The procedure has a relatively high complication rate, and is a very taxing procedure for the patient to undergo.

reports on edentulous jaws as opposed to reports on partially edentulous cases. Data could be extracted for block grafts and Le Fort I osteotomies but not, without knowledge of baseline defect characteristics, for other techniques like GBR, ridge splitting, or distraction osteogenesis.

Bone block grafting. Some scientific evidence supports the use of bone block grafts for vertical, horizontal, or combined augmentation of completely edentulous maxillae and mandibles presenting with severe resorption. Donor-site complications are documented in 8% to 11.1% and partial or complete graft loss in 8% to 20% of patients.

Le Fort I osteotomy. This maxillofacial procedure is widely used and supported by adequate evidence in the treatment of atrophic edentulous maxillae. It may be selected to deal with class IV, V, or VI atrophy (Cawood and Howell 1988) with the main objectives of achieving bone augmentation and three-dimensional repositioning of the maxilla to an ideal interarch relationship. An implant survival rate of 86.6% may be expected following this highly demanding surgical procedure.

All of the reported procedures for atrophic edentulous jaws (which could be assessed based on the inclusion criteria for this review) have yielded successful outcomes of augmentation. On the other hand, most of the authors of the included reports have provided scant information on pre- and postoperative ridge dimensions and the bone gains they achieved.

On balance, after reviewing the available literature there is no clearly identifiable criteria for selecting the type of augmentation technique to use for specific clinical situations in edentulous jaws. Decisions on which technique should be selected in specific edentulous situations continue to be guided by anecdotal evidence available to the clinician from experience and clinical training.

2.2.3 Patients with Completely Edentulous Jaws

Relatively few studies could be included that reported on bone augmentation in edentulous jaws. In most cases, it was impossible to distinguish data on completely edentulous jaws from data on partially edentulous jaws, since these patients groups were pooled in most relevant papers dealing with different surgical techniques.

Most authors disclosed neither pre- and postoperative ridge dimensions nor the bone gains achieved. As a result, broader selection criteria were used to include

2.3 References of the Systematic Review

For full citations, please consult the alphabetic list of references in Chapter 9.

Partially edentulous GBR with simultaneous implant placement
Dahlin and coworkers 1995; Fugazzotto 1997; Zitzmann and coworkers 1997; Peleg and coworkers 1999; von Arx and coworkers 1998; Lorenzoni and coworkers 1999; Carpio and coworkers 2000; Widmark and Ivanoff 2000; van Steenberghe and coworkers 2000; Nemcovsky and coworkers 2000; Blanco and coworkers 2005; De Boever and De Boever 2005; Hämmerle and coworkers 2008; Park and coworkers 2008; Jung and coworkers 2009; Dahlin and coworkers 2010.

Partially edentulous GBR with staged implant placement
Parodi and coworkers 1999; Chapasco and coworkers 1999; Meijndert and coworkers 2005; von Arx and Buser 2006; Geurs and coworkers 2008; Hämmerle and coworkers 2008.

Partially edentulous: block grafts for horizontal ridge augmentation
Buser and coworkers 1996; von Arx and coworkers 1998; Chiapasco and coworkers 1999; Acocella and coworkers 2010; Wallace and Gellin 2010; Cordaro and coworkers 2011b; Nissan and coworkers 2011.

Partially edentulous: ridge splitting/expansion for horizontal augmentation
Sethi and Kaus 2000; Chiapasco and coworkers 2006a; Blus and Szmukler-Moncler 2006; Gonzalez-Garcia and coworkers 2011; Anitua and coworkers 2011.

Partially edentulous with vertical defects: GBR with simultaneous implant placement
Simion and coworkers 2001; Simion and coworkers 2007; Llambes and coworkers 2007.

Partially edentulous with vertical defects: GBR with delayed implant placement
Simion and coworkers 2007; Todisco 2010.

Partially edentulous with vertical defects: treated with bone block grafts
Sethi and Kaus 2001; Bahat and Fontanessi 2001; Chiapasco and coworkers 2007b; Roccuzzo and coworkers 2007; Cordaro and coworkers 2010; Nissan and coworkers 2011.

Partially edentulous with vertical defects: treated with distraction osteogenesis
Gaggl and coworkers 2000; Rachmiel and coworkers 2001; Jensen and coworkers 2002; Chiapasco and coworkers 2004a; Marchetti and coworkers 2007; Chiapasco and coworkers 2007b; Robiony and coworkers 2008.

Edentulous: bone block grafts for vertical and/or horizontal bone augmentation
Adell and coworkers 1990; Jensen and Sindet-Pedersen 1991; Donovan and coworkers 1994; Triplett and Schow 1996; McGrath and coworkers 1996; Neyt and coworkers 1997; Lundgren and coworkers 1997; Schwartz-Arad and Lewin 2005; Smolka and coworkers 2006.

Edentulous: Le Fort I osteotomy and grafting for maxillary augmentation.
Isaksson and coworkers 1993; Li and coworkers 1996; Kahnberg and coworkers 1999; Stoelinga and coworkers 2000; Chiapasco and coworkers 2007a; De Santis and coworkers 2012.

3 Preoperative Assessment and Planning

L. Cordaro

3.1   Anatomy

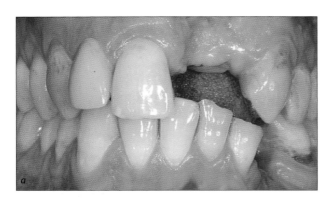

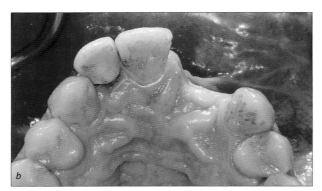

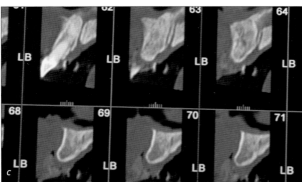

Any tooth loss may be followed by extensive resorption of the alveolar ridge. Due to the resulting bone loss, the alveolar anatomy will undergo various degrees of alteration.

Several authors have described this resorption process and suggested classifications defining different types of alveolar atrophy. A defect classification that gives consideration not only to anatomical features but also to available treatment options as proposed at the end of this chapter.

Staged procedures of augmenting the alveolar process are usually indicated in the presence of advanced bone resorption. This approach is not confined to specific jaw segments but may be performed anywhere in the mouth. Augmentation may be needed to insert implants of adequate dimensions or to create suitable conditions for an esthetic and functional implant-supported restoration. Requirements to achieve an "ideal" esthetic and functional outcome of prosthetic treatment include a correct interarch relationship, ideal soft-tissue support, and a reasonable height of the crowns involved in the planned prosthesis.

3.1.1   Bone Quality and Quantity for Implant Placement

Little research is available on how much bone is needed to safely insert an implant. It is mandatory, however, that implants be placed in the correct prosthodontic position according to the treatment plan. Frequently, there may be enough bone to place an implant but in a suboptimal position. Thus, ridges with sufficient bone volume may still need reconstruction to allow implants to be positioned correctly according to the restorative plan. (Figs 1a-c).

Figs 1a-c   Trauma case with loss of a central and a lateral maxillary incisor. A bony defect is clearly anticipated from the frontal and palatal clinical views (a, b). The crosssectional radiographic survey (c)[1] indicates that the residual crest is 7 mm wide and 14 mm high. While there is enough bone to place implants, this could only be achieved at the expense of suboptimal positioning. Given the esthetically sensitive location of the edentulous space, the only way to pursue a restoration-driven strategy of implant placement is to reconstruct the bone.

[1]TC reformatted with dentascan software.

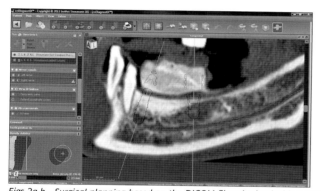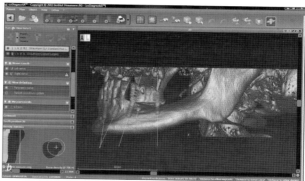

Figs 2a-b   Surgical planning based on the DICOM files obtained with a CBCT scan. In this particular case, only implants 6 mm in length can be placed above the alveolar nerve. The three-dimensional view permits an overall evaluation of the situation.

Reference must be made to guidelines that indicate the amount of bone required to insert the implants to their ideal positions. A good method of analyzing the dimensions of the defect is to use planning software in conjunction with three-dimensional images derived from cone-beam computed tomography (CBCT) scans (Figs 2a-b).

Alveolar bone width should exceed the diameter of the proposed implant by 1 to 1.5 mm both on the buccal and on the lingual or palatal side (Dietrich and coworkers 1993). Ridge width should be 6 to 7 mm for standard-diameter implants, 5 to 6 mm for reduced-diameter implants, and at least 7.5 mm for wide implants.

The amount of alveolar bone height required for long-term success of an implant-supported restoration has been widely discussed. Some authors in the early history of osseointegrated implants would claim that long implants were required to engage the cortical bone at the apex and neck. Today it is clear, however, that similar success rates are achieved with micro-rough-surface implants 8 mm (mandible) or 10 mm (maxilla) in length (Buser 1997). Several recent authors have devoted great attention to the outcomes of shorter implants 6 mm in length and have presented encouraging results from studies performed in controlled environments (Annibali and coworkers 2012; Atieh and coworkers 2012; Sun and coworkers 2011; Telleman and coworkers 2011).

Even though unsupported by strong evidence, the use of short implants to support very long crowns may lead to suboptimal esthetic results and jeopardize long-term outcomes. On the other hand, standard-diameter 6mm implants may be planned if the interocclusal space is maintained or reduced. The use of short and wide implants may be associated with difficulties in achieving primary implant stability.

Aside from bone quantity, another important consideration in dealing with alveolar atrophy is bone quality, which may affect the primary implant stability essential to osseointegration. Local jawbone will usually exhibit a similar degree of quality at the alveolar and basal bone levels. As a general rule, maxillary bone is softer and less dense than mandibular bone and has a favorable blood supply to facilitate healing of grafts and implants.

Conversely, mandibular bone will usually offer higher density and a cortical component of substantial thickness. Although there is little scientific evidence to confirm this statement, the reduced vascularization offered by cortical bone may affect the healing properties of grafts. The cancellous component of the mandible, notably in the anterior region between the mental foramina, may almost disappear as resorption progresses to extreme atrophy. This point must be considered very carefully from a surgical viewpoint. There is a risk of overheating the bone while preparing the implant bed or inserting the implant. Measures must be taken to avoid the deleterious effects of such overheating on implant integration by using sharp drills at reduced speed, using copious irrigation with saline, guiding the handpiece with a light touch to reduce pressure, and tapping of the bone prior to implant insertion.

3.1.2   Resorption Patterns in the Edentulous Maxilla and Mandible

Different patterns of resorption are seen in the maxilla and mandible. Tooth loss in maxillary anterior and posterior segments is followed by resorption of the alveolar bone toward the midline, which causes reductions in the transverse and sagittal arch dimensions in addition to a reduction in alveolar height. As a result, atrophic edentulous maxillae are normally characterized by narrower and shorter dimensions of the alveolar bone than in their original dentate state. Depending on the degree of atrophy, even the basal bone may be affected.

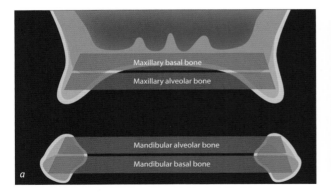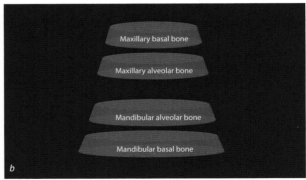

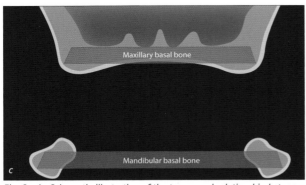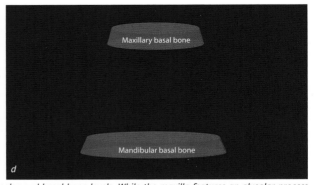

Figs 3a-d   Schematic illustration of the transversal relationship between alveolar and basal bone levels. While the maxilla features an alveolar process wider than the basal bone, the reverse is true of the mandible. As a consequence, resorption of alveolar bone will usually give rise to a transverse and sagittal discrepancy between both atrophic jaws.

These relationships between the maxilla and mandible can be illustrated by two schematic cones tapering from bottom to top (Figs 3a-d). Thus, partial or complete resorption of the alveolar process will greatly impact the interarch relationship not only in the vertical plane but also in the transverse and sagittal planes. Complete edentulism with advanced resorption in both jaws will commonly involve a large discrepancy between both basal bones, mimicking a class III malocclusion with sagittal and transverse discrepancies.

In the mandible, the basal bone is wider than the alveolar process, and bone resorption after tooth loss occurs in the direction of the vestibule. As a consequence, vertical bone loss increases the width of the mandibular arch. Moreover, the anteroposterior dimensions of the edentulous mandible are also increased due to the fact that the basal bone of the symphysis is more anterior than the respective alveolar bone.

In partially edentulous patients with advanced resorption, it is crucial to understand the typical resorption pattern of the alveolar process. Reconstruction of lost bone should reverse the path of the resorption process to restore the anatomical situation before the start of the resorption process. The resorption pattern has important clinical implications for various aspects of the treatment of alveolar atrophies.

Horizontal defects are usually treated with augmentation in the buccal direction. This can be achieved with different grafting techniques. Buccal augmentation is frequently adequate in maxillary defects in anterior and premolar areas where resorption occurs towards the palate. Buccal augmentation, however, may cause suboptimal outcomes in the posterior mandible by overexpansion of the alveolar crest. This may result in the final coronal position of the implant neck being too far buccally, mimicking a posterior cross-bite situation.

3.1.3 Bone Situation at Adjacent Teeth

The anatomy of the defect has to be evaluated not only in relation to the type of resorption (horizontal, vertical, or combined) or to the size of the defect (volume of lost bone), but also in relation to the neighboring teeth.

Both the residual dentition adjacent to the edentulous space to be reconstructed and the anatomy of the adjacent bone are important in assessing the defect and the appropriate reconstruction strategy.

The periodontal attachment level, the interproximal bony peaks, and the width of buccal bone covering the roots adjacent to the missing tooth or teeth have to be carefully evaluated.

For a vertical reconstruction, the interproximal bony peak of the tooth adjacent to the defect represents the most coronal level that may be achieved (Fig. 4). It may be assumed that if a vertical bone graft is placed more coronally than the bony peak of the adjacent tooth, resorption of the graft will occur or a vertical periodontal defect will be created because it is not possible to create a new periodontal attachment at the level of the grafted bone (Fig 4). A vertical graft exceeding this level can be expected to undergo resorption or to involve a periodontal defect, considering that new periodontal attachment cannot form between the tooth and grafted bone.

For horizontal bone reconstruction, the amount of alveolar bone covering the buccal aspect of the adjacent tooth needs to be considered. Evaluating this parameter correctly is essential to the assessment of horizontal defects.

In edentulous gaps with horizontal resorption, the buccal bone covering the remaining mesial and distal roots identifies the so-called "bony alveolar envelope." When mesial and distal horizontal bone support is present, the defect may be considered a "hole" in the alveolar ridge, and a favorable healing pattern can be anticipated for the bone reconstruction. This is due to increased soft-tissue support, which reduces pressure on the reconstructed site during healing and provides a greater contact area between the graft and the recipient site (Fig 5). Conversely, thin buccal bone at adjacent teeth, missing distal teeth, or extended dental gaps create an anatomical situation in which the bone has to be rebuilt "outside of the bony envelope" (Fig 5). This is accompanied by reduced soft-tissue support, reduced vascularization, and reduced graft contact with the recipient site (Fig 6).

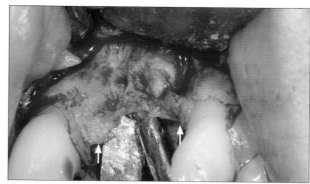

Fig 4   In evaluating this pure vertical defect at the site of a missing central incisor, the vertical level of the bony peaks is paramount. The mesial peak adjacent to the residual central incisor is more favorable than the one adjacent to the lateral incisor. (Please note the arrows indicating the two interproximal bony peaks).

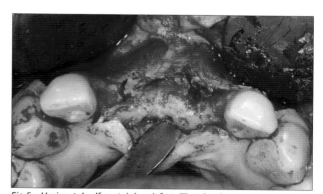

Fig 5   Horizontal self-containing defect. The alveolar structure of the adjacent lateral incisors will offer support for the reconstruction. In this clinical situation, it may be sufficient to use particulated graft material with membrane protection in a staged surgical approach.

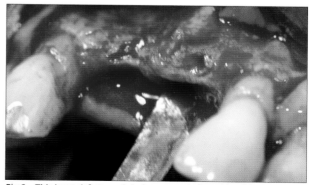

Fig 6   This bone defect needs to be augmented outside of the bony envelope. Since the adjacent bone structure does not offer horizontal support for the reconstruction, a technique should be used that includes space-creating effects.

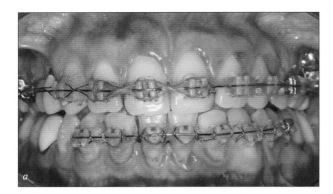
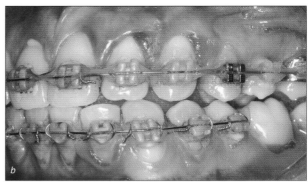

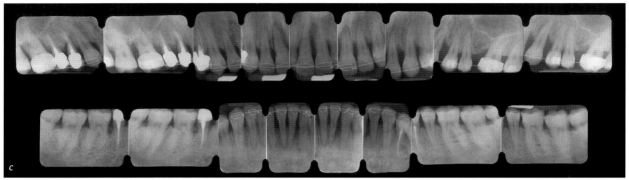

Figs 7a-c   In this patient, orthodontic treatment was conducted in the presence of uncontrolled periodontal disease, aggravating the clinical situation. Tooth mobility increased, and plaque control was lacking.

3.1.4   Periodontal Evaluation of Adjacent Teeth

Another parameter to be evaluated is the periodontal attachment levels of any teeth adjacent to the defect. In patients affected by periodontal disease, it is mandatory that implant placement be planned only after effective treatment of the active periodontal lesions with the aid of hygienic and potentially surgical periodontal therapy (either resective or regenerative). This also applies to deficient ridges that require staged reconstruction. Figures 7 and 8 illustrate the clinical case of an adult patient who had undergone orthodontic treatment to correct tooth migration secondary to non-diagnosed periodontal disease. In patients with active periodontal lesions, orthodontic treatment accelerates bone disruption. In this patient, tooth 11 had to be extracted after active periodontal treatment, followed by staged bone augmentation.

Any vertical periodontal defects that may be associated with teeth adjacent to the deficient alveolar segment need to be carefully assessed. No evidence is available about the outcomes of reconstructing adjacent periodontal defects simultaneously with bone defects.

A think mucosa, often referred to as a thick periodontal or gingival biotype is valuable in achieving an effective staged reconstruction. A thin mucosa may predispose to soft-tissue recession at adjacent teeth or soft-tissue dehiscences of the wound. Thin and highly scalloped biotypes will require more attention in designing the flap and positioning the vertical releasing incisions. In some cases, and notably in the esthetic zone, it is advisable to use a wider flap with only one distal releasing incision. This helps reduce the risk of recession in the esthetic zone.

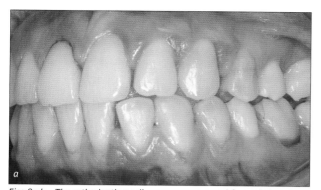 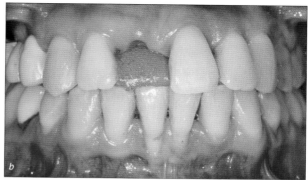

Figs 8a-b   The orthodontic appliances were removed for periodontal treatment. Tooth 21 was extracted. Only when the periodontal disease was under control and tooth mobility had decreased could an implant-supported single-tooth restoration be planned.

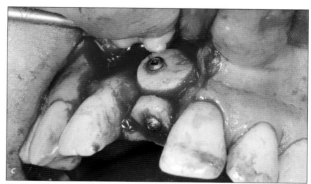

Fig 8c   The thin periodontal biotype and the need for augmentation outside of the bony envelope—due to reduced horizontal bone support—made a block graft necessary in this specific patient.

3.1.5   Anatomical Limitations and Risks

Staged jaw reconstructions should only be performed by surgeons with an in-depth knowledge of maxillary and mandibular anatomy and anatomical relationships. Although subject to similar anatomical limitations as implant surgery, reconstructive surgery will usually require more extensive dissection and broader exposure of adjacent structures. The surgeon must undertake a careful preoperative assessment of the local anatomy, including the site to be augmented and its related structures, and the anatomy of potential donor sites for bone harvesting.

While a detailed description of atrophic jaw anatomy is beyond the scope of this volume, relevant anatomical landmarks will be discussed selectively in connection with the various surgical approaches. Some interventions—such as Le Fort I osteotomies or extraoral bone harvesting—require in-depth knowledge of the anatomy of the maxillofacial region or extra-oral parts of the body, such as the iliac crest or the calvaria, which are not usually associated with dental procedures. These operations are performed by maxillofacial surgeons, but will be described in this book since they are needed, in selected cases, to achieve effective reconstruction of the jaws in preparation for implant placement and delivery of an implant-supported restoration.

3.2 Medical History

Any patient who is a candidate for an implant-supported restoration should undergo a thorough medical evaluation. This is also true of patients who need a bone reconstruction of the alveolus in preparation for implant placement. When a staged reconstruction is needed, the surgery is generally more complicated than implant placement in sites with adequate bone volume. At least two surgical sessions are required, the first to perform the augmentation procedure and the second to place the implants. The first stage will usually involve the harvesting of bone, which often means that a second surgical site is needed. Obviously, the health situation of these patients should be evaluated not only in relation to procedures and potential complications but also to determine whether the patients are fit enough for extensive surgery. Alternatives such as restorations not supported by implants should be considered if relevant health problems are identified.

Two different perspectives should be considered in evaluating the medical history and current health situation of each patient:

* Risk factors jeopardizing the success of surgical and restorative treatment.
* Systemic conditions involving an increased risk of medical complications.

3.2.1   Risk Factors Jeopardizing the Success of Surgical and Restorative Treatment

An ITI consensus paper (Bornstein and coworkers 2009) assessed risk factors in dental implant therapy. Several diseases and treatment modalities were analyzed for the risk they may pose to long-term implant success, including Sjögren's syndrome, lichen ruber planus, HIV infection, ectodermal dysplasia, Parkinson's disease, immunosuppression after organ transplantation, cardiovascular disease, Crohn's disease, diabetes, osteoporo-

sis, oral bisphosphonate medication, and radiotherapy to treat head-andneck malignancies. Any absolute or relative contraindications to implant therapy associated with most of these situations were found to be based on low-level evidence.

There is more data available in the literature regarding the influence of diabetes, osteoporosis, bisphosphonate therapy, radiotherapy, smoking, and a history of periodontitis on the outcome of implant therapy. A brief overview of the evidence for these conditions follows.

Diabetes
While diabetes used to be considered a potential risk factor to the long-term survival and success of oral implants, recent reviews have failed to establish an unequivocal correlation between diabetes and long-term implant success.

Several studies actually did show higher failure rates in diabetic patients, but it has been impossible to demonstrate a clearly detrimental effect of the disease on long-term implant success (Bornstein and coworkers 2009). This does not change the fact that the presence of diabetes requires close attention prior to planning reconstructive surgery. As uncontrolled diabetes is capable of seriously affecting wound healing, reconstructive surgery must not be considered in diabetic patients unless the disease is under control. It is therefore advisable to consult with an endocrinologist if there is any evidence of unstable disease.

Osteoporosis
Several studies have investigated associations between osteoporosis and implant failure. There is evidence that implants placed in osteoporotic patients have clinical outcomes similar to those in control patients (Bornstein and coworkers 2009). No significant relationships was found between success/survival rates and histories of chronic corticosteroid use (potentially reducing the mineral content of bone) or hormone-replacement therapy

for osteoporosis prevention (Steiner and Ramp 1990). The more significant clinical issue is when the patient with osteoporosis is being managed with bisphosphonate therapy (Wang and coworkers 2007).

Bisphosphonate therapy

Bisphosphonates reduce the activity of osteoclasts. They were introduced to treat severe diseases, such as multiple myeloma or bone metastases from malignant neoplasm. These drugs are usually administered intravenously at high doses. In 2003 it was reported and demonstrated that bisphosphonate-related osteonecrosis of the jaws (BRONJ) frequently occurs after tooth extraction in patients who are being treated with i.v. bisphosphonates (Marx 2003). It is considered inappropriate to perform bone augmentation under these circumstances.

Lower-dose oral bisphosphonates are used in the treatment of osteoporosis or Paget's disease. There is limited evidence from the literature as to complications or implant failure in patients thus treated (Wang and coworkers 2007). Oral bisphosphonates should be considered a potential risk factor for osteonecrosis of the jaw but not for implant success and survival per se (Grant and coworkers 2008; Kumar and Honne 2012).

Radiotherapy

Radiation therapy is commonly used in the treatment of head and neck cancers, very often as one element of combined regimens that also involve surgery and chemotherapy.

The task of identifying any effects of radiotherapy on implant treatment is complicated by different irradiation protocols used in different clinical situations and by the fact that most patients with malignancies will usually exhibit other potential risk factors as well. In addition, situations vary with regard to the radiation fields and dosages, whether radiotherapy is applied prior to implant placement, immediately thereafter, or after diagnosing a tumor when oral implants have long been in function. Many of the available studies on the subject were performed against the background of different clinical situations that cannot be readily compared (Colella and coworkers 2007). It is difficult to draw conclusions about any effects that radiotherapy may have on surgical jaw reconstruction or implant placement.

There are reports on osteoradionecrosis and soft-tissue dehiscence in previously irradiated patients undergoing oral surgery. Some authors have demonstrated increased failure rates, notably in the maxilla, whereas others found no statistical association of this type (Colella and coworkers 2007).

Hyperbaric oxygen therapy (HBO) has been advocated to improve bone and soft-tissue healing after implant or reconstructive surgery in patients with a history of radiotherapy. A beneficial effect of this measure is difficult to identify based on data from the literature (Esposito and coworkers 2008). As a rule, patients undergoing radiotherapy should be treated in centers experienced in treating and rehabilitating patients with these particular clinical problems.

In fact, resective surgery often ends up being used in clinical situations where prosthetic treatment may be complicated, and the use of implants may improve the final outcome of the restoration. On the other hand, complications related to surgical treatment of irradiated jaws may be very serious.

Smoking

Smoking is known to reduce the wound-healing capacity. The habit also affects the progression of periodontitis and carries an increased risk of peri-implant disease and the loss of dental implants. The latter was clearly demonstrated and discussed in a systematic review published after the 4th ITI Consensus Conference in Stuttgart, Germany (Heitz-Mayfield and Huynh-Ba 2009). Staged augmentation procedures should be planned with a view to the fact that they carry a higher risk in smokers than non-smokers.

Periodontitis

Lower implant success rates are found in patients with a history of periodontitis than in other patients. Implant treatment may be considered after periodontal disease has been treated, controlled by adequate hygiene, and followed up by a careful maintenance program, although the risk of peri-implant complications will still be increased in this situation. As stated, active periodontal lesions like deep pockets should be treated and controlled well before considering implant or staged jaw reconstruction surgery (Heitz-Mayfield and Huynh-Ba 2009). An even higher risk of implant failure and peri-implant disease is present in smokers with a history of periodontitis. These risks should be carefully evaluated and discussed with the patient before embarking on any complex treatments such as those involving staged reconstruction of jawbone (Heitz-Mayfield and Huynh-Ba 2009).

3.2.2 Systemic Conditions Involving an Increased Risk of Medical Complications

Any medical treatment must be preceded by an evaluation of the patient's general health; reconstructive bone surgery prior to dental implant placement is no exception. General contraindications to oral surgery include uncontrolled diabetes, recent (less than 3 months) myocardial infarction, or severe liver disease with impaired hepatic function.

A number of relevant medical conditions are routinely controlled with drugs whose action may interfere with the mechanisms of soft- and hard-tissue healing. Careful attention is needed in patients treated with corticosteroids, antirheumatic immunosappressive drugs, anticoagulants, or concomitant chemotherapy. Anticoagulant therapy should be adjusted before the surgical session, and surgery must be postponed in patients currently undergoing chemotherapy against malignancies.

In patients with compromised general health or life-threatening systemic disease, no bone reconstruction should be performed before the medical condition has stabilized and improved.

There is a need to weigh up the risk of general medical complications in patients needing a staged alveolar bone reconstruction against alternative non-implant treatment options.

Edentulous patients with atrophic jaws are often elderly and frail, suffering from cardiac or vascular conditions or other chronic diseases, which are usually controlled by medications. Patients with effectively controlled and stable disease may still be good candidates for staged jawbone reconstruction. With optimal management, a chronic systemic condition may remain stable for numerous years. In evaluating patients of this kind, the risks of reconstructive surgery should be related to the many years of improved oral function that an implant-supported restoration may offer. It may be useful in these situations to select a mode of implant treatment that will offer a reduced level of surgical invasiveness. An overdenture, for example, may require fewer implants than a full-arch fixed prosthesis.

3.3 Clinical Examination and Planning Aids

A comprehensive clinical examination is mandatory whenever an implant reconstruction is planned, and this stage would be incomplete without taking advantage of radiographic techniques and other planning aids. Also, there may be a need to seek expert opinions from other specialists like an endodontist or orthodontist. Information collected during the initial clinical examination and the result of correct prosthetic planning are the most important factors in developing the final treatment plan.

A number of parameters need to be evaluated during the clinical examination:

- Soft-tissue situation in the area to be treated and adjacent to areas.
- Overall periodontal health, oral hygiene, and patient compliance.
- Periodontal, endodontic, and reconstructive state of any adjacent teeth.
- Function and prognosis of the opposing dentition, including its interarch relationship in the frontal, sagittal and transverse planes.
- Interdental space.
- A careful clinical examination may also give some information on ridge width.

Great attention should be devoted to evaluating the soft tissues, since this aspect is highly important. The success of most of the surgical techniques described in this volume depends on stable soft-tissue closure at the time of bone reconstruction for primary wound healing over the reconstructed site. Soft-tissue quality and quantity make an impact on surgical outcomes. Other soft-tissue-related variables include the surgical approach taken and the surgeon's expertise and experience. A wide band of keratinized tissue at the incision line will assist the surgeon in managing the surgical flaps. Though not formally demonstrated, it is generally believed that thick soft tissues are more resistant to suture or flap dehiscences.

The patient's overall periodontal situation needs to be evaluated to make sure that no active deep periodontal pockets are present before a staged reconstruction is planned. Oral hygiene and compliance should be evaluated. It should be understood that complex surgical and prosthetic treatments should only be performed in patients who clearly understand the role of plaque control in the maintenance phase subsequent to active treatment.

The first patient visit is devoted to establishing the general prosthetic needs and discussing them with the patient. This is a mandatory step in edentulous patients, given that there are different possible prosthetic solutions that involve different strategies of implant placement.

While the clinical examination may offer preliminary information about the interdental space and interarch relationship, it is recommended to obtain study casts with a diagnostic wax-up for evaluation and discussion with the patient during the second visit. In edentulous patients, considerable attention should be devoted at this point to the facial profile and the soft-tissue support needed to achieve an acceptable outcome. The planned height of the lower third of the face also has to be evaluated. Care should be taken to document all relevant aspects pertaining to facial appearance and soft-tissue assessment. Extra and intraoral photographs are an invaluable aid in developing the final treatment plan.

The patient's expectations should be discussed prior to drawing up a preliminary restorative plan.

In cases requiring a cross-sectional radiographic evaluation, a radiographic stent is derived from the diagnostic wax-up for use during the examination.

3.3.1 Study Casts and Diagnostic Wax-Up

A comprehensive dental examination is always carried out as a preliminary diagnostic phase in these cases; usually a plain radiograph, such as an orthopanoramic radiograph, is available. Study casts help to provide a more precise diagnosis and are an invaluable aid in the design of the definitive treatment plan. A wax-up of the planned final restoration helps clarify the amount of soft tissue support needed to achieve a prosthetic result that mimics the natural dentition.

This diagnostic wax-up also supports the process of deciding on the type and design of the final restoration. For example, there are three alternative methods of correcting alveolar bone resorption in edentulous patients: by reconstructing and repositioning bone, by using pink acrylic or porcelain on a fixed restoration, or via the flange of an overdenture. One of these options should be selected after discussing them with the patient aided by the diagnostic wax-up.

The next step is to determine the need for cross-sectional radiographic assessment.

3.3.2 Radiographic Examination and Planning

Radiographic images are always necessary in implant dentistry. Periapical radiographs, orthopanoramic views, and lateral cephalometric views of the skull are the standard examinations for implant diagnostics and treatment planning. Orthopantomograms and periapical radiographs are routinely used in partially edentulous patients because they readily yield information about adjacent and opposing teeth and vertical bone quantity, even though the ridge dimensions cannot be accurately measured. Further insights into ridge width may be gained by the clinical examination and additional radiographs if indicated.

Frequently, situations of this type will require cross-sectional imaging to precisely assess horizontal and vertical ridge dimensions, bony support available from adjacent teeth, and the presence of any ongoing inflammatory processes in the sinus membrane.

In edentulous patients, basic information about residual jaw anatomy can be obtained via orthopantomograms and lateral cephalograms. These will allow the surgeon to evaluate ridge height and the presence of pathologic lesions. They may also disclose vertical deficits under the nasal or sinus floor and distal to the mental foramina, allowing the surgeon to detect areas of reduced height in these jaw segments but not to measure them precisely.

Again, the usual suggestion is to perform a cross-sectional radiographic examination when some degree of bone atrophy is expected in edentulous cases.

Although several different technologies of cross-sectional radiography are available, cone-beam computed tomography (CBCT) is currently the most widely used version in implant dentistry. Its popularity results from the high precision it offers and its reduced doses of radiation compared to other techniques. Before the introduction of CBCT, examinations of this type used to be performed on CT scans reformatted with dental software.

Conventional CT scans are not recommended for routine application in the kind of examinations here discussed, since they expose patients to substantially higher levels of radiation than CBCT scans. Also, radiation doses are known to differ not only between CT and CBCT but also between CBCT scanners from different manufacturers. It is important to know which scanner will be used before referring a patient to a radiologist.

Another recommendation is to use a radiographic stent during scanning, which may include one or more radiopaque references in accordance with the planned prosthetic elements, offering a direct and instant way of relating tooth positions to residual bone structures.

Using advanced planning software, implants and potential abutments can today be planned and inserted to their desired positions in three-dimensional virtual environments, allowing any bone volumes for augmentation to be evaluated before the actual surgical procedure. Originally designed for guided implant placement, these software applications are also effective in conducting presurgical assessments of reconstructive strategies or bone graft volumes, and they can be used to create precise stereolithographic jaw replicas (these are potentially very helpful in presurgical planning). Some authors have advocated a strategy whereby blocks of bone substitute are adapted to the stereolithographic model and then sterilized for use as custom grafts during reconstructive surgery (Edwards 2010).

3.4 Alternatives to Staged Augmentation

There are several alternatives to staged jaw augmentation in preparation for implant treatment, all of which should be carefully evaluated and discussed with the patient:

- Removable dentures
- Tooth-supported fixed prostheses
- Prosthetic-compensation solutions, either in the form of elongated teeth or by adding pink acrylic or porcelain to compensate for lost soft-tissue structures
- Short or narrow implants with or without a prosthetic compromise
- Bone augmentation performed simultaneously with implant placement

Removable dentures. May be considered in patients with budget constraints or seriously impaired general health. As noted before, systemic health may be compromised notably in elderly edentulous patients. The advantages of an implant-supported restoration and the impact on the patient's quality of life should, however, be carefully evaluated to determine whether the risk involved in implant surgery is acceptable.

Tooth-supported fixed prostheses. These are typically indicated when dealing with posterior bone deficiencies in edentulous spaces of one or two missing teeth if adjacent teeth are present and have been, or are planned to be, restored. They may overcome the need for a bone reconstruction without further damage to the teeth that have already been restored or where a restoration is indicated. A tooth-supported fixed prosthesis should be considered in any situation that involves a deficient residual ridge in the presence of neighboring teeth intended to be restored.

Prosthetic-compensation solutions. These options may reduce the need for surgical augmentation, though normally at the expense of optimal outcomes. Pink acrylic or porcelain is capable of solving a variety of esthetic problems associated with ridge atrophy by masking areas of hard-/soft-tissue loss and allowing for a prosthesis with ideally sized and positioned teeth.

Several technical problems may be encountered. While it is extremely difficult to match the original color of a patient's soft tissues, it may be impossible to effectively hide the transition zone from the tissues to the pink material, especially in the partially edentulous situation. Restorations with a pink component should not be used in patients with a high smile line (exposing entire crowns during function and smiling). Yet they are often utilized in medium- and low smile-line cases. They commonly used in the mandible and in edentulous patients. The cleansability of such structures should be respected, especially when they are applied in a ridge-lap fashion.

Short or narrow implants. These options may be considered in cases with reduced bone volume. Today's standards require that implants supporting a restoration should guarantee an ideal esthetic outcome, which can only be achieved if the final restoration is similar to the natural dentition with regard to tooth size and position and soft-tissue contour. Good soft-tissue support requires an adequate bone volume. Reduced-diameter implants should be only considered if an ideal (prosthetically guided) three-dimensional implant position can be achieved.

Some situations may suggest the use of reduced-diameter implants, such as when an overdenture or splinting of narrow implants is planned, or when reduced diameter implants can be splinted with standard-diameter implants. Notably those with an internal connection design have a weak point at the level of the implant-abutment interface and may be prone to fracture. A stronger Ti-Zr alloy was recently introduced to overcome this risk (Gottlow and coworkers 2012). Narrow implants of this novel type may be used with greater confidence, although some limitations still apply, including their use for single-molar replacement or as distal abutment supporting a cantilever. Ti-Zr implants are available both as soft tissue- and as bone-level implants.

Short implants may be used above the maxillary sinus floor or the mandibular alveolar canal. They are an acceptable solution in these situations if adequate tooth dimensions can still be achieved. As several studies have demonstrated acceptable success and survival rates of short implants, these should be considered a viable option in some situations (Annibali and coworkers 2011; Sun and coworkers 2011).

Furthermore, it should be pointed out that any need for extensive lower-jaw reconstruction in elderly edentulous patients is seriously called into question by the fact that atrophic edentulous mandibles can be effectively restored with an overdenture retained by short interforaminal implants (Stellingsma and coworkers 2005).

Bone augmentation simultaneously with implant placement. Unlike other alternatives to staged jaw reconstruction in preparation for implant placement, this approach will allow implants to be inserted to their ideal positions (Buser and coworkers 2004). Usually, the simultaneous approach is accomplished by guided bone regeneration (GBR). It is advantageous by reducing surgical sessions and, potentially, by creating space via the inserted implants during maturation of the bone graft. GBR may be provided with different bone grafts or substitutes, different barrier membranes, and one-piece (soft-tissue-level) or two-piece (bone-level) implants.

Resorbable membranes are easier to use and will offer uneventful healing even on becoming mildly exposed. Non-resorbable membranes—expanded polytetrafluoroethylene (e-PTFE) is the predominant material—have yielded excellent results in the hands of experts and offer the best performance in terms of bone growth, provided that soft-tissue healing is achieved and maintained during graft maturation. On the downside, premature exposure of a non-resorbable membrane may necessitate its removal along with the graft and the implant.

Simultaneous procedures of GBR and implant placement have proven effective in selected clinical situations, notably for bone augmentation in single-tooth edentulous spaces (Yildirim and coworkers 1997). Combined with transmucosal healing, they can minimize surgical steps and patient morbidity (Cordaro and coworkers 2012b). Simultaneous GBR, however, may not be appropriate in all clinical situations. Before the introduction of CT and CBCT scanners for pretreatment use, the decision to perform GBR simultaneously with implant placement could only be made at the time of surgery following flap reflection and direct inspection of the existing bone morphology. Often the intended strategy had to be changed in favor of a staged approach if the bone volume was found to be inadequate during the procedure. Today's diagnostic tools are more advanced, allowing surgeons to anticipate more confidently whether a simultaneous or staged approach should be taken.

Despite careful planning, there may still be occasional situations in which a surgical plan needs to be changed from simultaneous to staged augmentation after flap elevation.

3.4.1 Type of Edentulism and Defect Type

Staged jawbone reconstruction may be required in a variety of clinical situations and are associated with different problems and challenges. The procedures involved will be grouped into different categories for better understanding of their respective treatment rationales.

The subsequent chapters of this book will shed light on these reconstructive procedures based on different types of edentulism, including single-tooth gaps, extended edentulous spaces with multiple missing teeth (which may or may not involve a distal free-end situation) or completely edentulous situations in at least one jaw.

Each category will be further subdivided into defect types, including horizontal, vertical, and combined defects (Table 1 and Fig 9). This subdivision is made for practical clinical reasons, considering that different treatment strategies may be needed to deal with different defects and clinical situations. A more detailed discussion is provided in Chapter 4.12.

As noted previously, conventional alternatives of non-implant prosthetic treatment are available in all of these clinical situations. While these non-implant options should often be considered as second rather than first choice due to their suboptimal functional and/or esthetic outcomes, they should still receive due consideration in the planning stage with a view to cost, simplicity, patient compliance, and patient health.

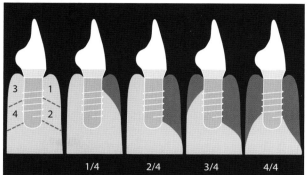

Fig 9 Classification of alveolar bone defects by Terheyden (2010), defining the typical pattern of resorption that an alveolar crest will undergo in the wake of tooth extraction. Defect types are grouped into four quarters that relate the amount of existing bone loss to the position of a prospective dental implant. In the initial phase of resorption, the facial bone plate is reduced to less than 50% of the prospective implant length; defects of this type in single-tooth gaps are typically contained and are referred to as dehiscence defects when an implant is already present (1/4). Continued buccal resorption will then create a knife-edge narrow ridge that is not yet reduced in height while showing a buccal wall reduced to more than 50% of the prospective implant length (2/4). It will normally take years for tooth loss to result in partial (3/4) and finally complete (4/4) height reduction of the ridge via resorption of its oral component.

Table 1 Overview of defect types.

Defect type	Single-tooth gap	Extended edentulous space, free-end situation	Completely edentulous jaw
1/4	Dehiscence defect, self-containing	Multiple dehiscence defects, self-containing	Multiple dehiscence defects, self-containing
2/4	Horizontal defect, non-self-containing, requires augmentation outside the existing bony envelope	Horizontal defect, non-self-containing, requires augmentation outside the existing bony envelope	Knife-edge ridge
3/4	Combined horizontal and vertical defect	Combined horizontal and vertical defect	Vertically reduced knife-edge ridge (Cawood class IV)
4/4	Through-and-through defect	Strictly vertical defect	Total jaw atrophy (Cawood classes V and VI)

The following is an overview of key parameters to be assessed in each clinical case:

Single-tooth gaps:
- Visible or nonvisible in the patient's smile
- Vertical position of interproximal bony peaks
- Soft-tissue thickness (thick, medium, thin)
- Tooth shape (triangular, rectangular)
- Presence of keratinized mucosa
- Defect type (vertical, horizontal, combined)
- Status of adjacent teeth (intact, periodontally compromised, restored, failing restoration)

Extended edentulous spaces:
- Visible or nonvisible in the patient's smile
- Vertical position of interproximal bony peaks at adjacent teeth
- Soft-tissue thickness (thick, medium, thin)
- Presence of keratinized mucosa
- Defect type (vertical, horizontal, combined)
- Status of maxillary sinus (presence or absence of pathology or septa)
- Interarch relationship (reduced or increased vertical space)

Completely edentulous jaws:
- Opposing dentition
- Vertical interarch relationship (reduced or increased space)
- Horizontal or transverse interarch relationship
- Status of maxillary sinus (presence or absence of pathology or septa)
- Presence or absence of keratinized mucosa

In addition to types of edentulism, the surgical rationale proposed in this textbook is also based on a classification of defect types. The following table will be used as a schematic guide to suggest the viable treatment options in the clinical cases.

4 Methods for Ridge Augmentation

H. Terheyden, L. Cordaro

A need for ridge augmentation arises whenever the existing bone volume of an atrophic ridge would otherwise be insufficient for ideal implant placement. The various methods available for ridge augmentation will be discussed in this chapter.

4.1 The GBR Principle

Guided bone regeneration (GBR) refers to the use of barrier membranes in the treatment of alveolar-ridge defects. Another term describing this method is "membrane-protected bone regeneration" (Bosshard and Schenk 2010). A barrier membrane is used to separate the tissue compartment made up of bone, its adjacent marrow cavity, and the bone defect from the overlying soft tissues. Coverage by this barrier will allow the defect volume to be populated with new blood vessels and osteogenic cells from the bone-marrow cavity and the bone surface. The latter is usually facilitated by perforation of the cortical plate of the underlying bone unless the bone bleeds spontaneously (as in fresh extraction sockets). Cell occlusiveness is not required for a membrane to offer a barrier function (Mardas and coworkers 2003).

However, there is more to a membrane than its separating barrier effect. A membrane will also stabilize the blood coagulum and any particulated grafting materials underneath. A membrane also offers protection against premature osteoclastic surface resorption by blocking the pathway for blood-borne osteoclast precursor cells from the overlying soft tissues until neovascularization takes place under the membrane from the defect side and later, after a few weeks, through the resorbable membrane. Finally, a soft membrane material has a bolstering effect and protects the overlying soft-tissue flap from sharp edges of bone blocks or other biomaterials.

In staged procedures of alveolar grafting, GBR is used for both horizontal and vertical augmentation. After wide flap elevation and perforation of the pristine crest, the graft material is applied and covered by a membrane. As resorbable collagen membrane loses its barrier function within the relatively short period of several weeks, a double-layer technique (Fig 1) has been recommended to ensure a prolonged barrier function (Bosshard and Schenk 2010). Pins may be used to secure the membrane, although they are not usually required with soft collagen membranes.

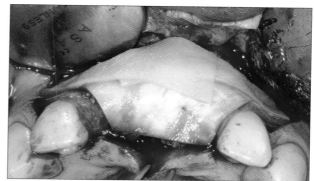

Fig 1   Resorbable collagen membrane placed in a double-layer technique (possibly using a third layer in the central portion) for a prolonged barrier function.

Several methods can be used to create more space, if needed, for staged augmentation in defects that are not self-containing. One example would be to use non-resorbable membranes that are reinforced by titanium structures incorporated during manufacture. Other options include the use of tenting pins and screws to support the membrane. Resorbable collagen membranes, by contrast, are soft and will collapse into the defect unless evenly supported across the defect, which is usually accomplished with bone substitute as filler. Since bone substitutes are not by themselves osteoinductive, they are normally combined with autologous bone grafts in mixed (composite) form. A layered technique can be

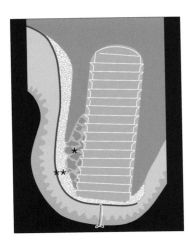

Fig 2 Layered concept of bone augmentation: bone chips (*), bone substitute (**), and collagen membrane (blue line).

applied by placing autologous bone chips where total bone regeneration is mandatory (e.g. at the prospective implant site) followed by placing bone substitutes into areas where the aim is to provide contour augmentation (Fig 2; Buser and coworkers 2008). In large defects that are not self-containing and that require a highly predictable bone volume, bone block grafts can be used to stabilize the membrane-protected defect volume.

4.2 Flap Design and Surgical Access for Ridge Augmentation

In general, the most appropriate surgical access for ridge augmentation is provided by midcrestal incisions over the edentulous space and sulcular incisions around teeth, followed by elevation of a fullthickness mucoperiosteal flap (Figs 3a-d). The main advantage of these incision lines is that they preserve (rather than sever) the pathways of natural blood vessels and nerve supply inside the flap. Extracted teeth leave behind a rather poorly vascularized area in the middle of the crest, known as the "mucosal linea alba". This line is located within keratinized mucosa and is a good place for an incision. Neither sulcular nor midcrestal incisions will result in any visible scars. They do leave behind intact soft tissue for revision surgery that may become necessary in the future. Predictable wound closure through rapid healing and regeneration of the junctional epithelium is another benefit offered by these incisions. Also, extension of the flap if required is a relatively straightforward maneuver. Other advantages include minimal bleeding in the subperiosteal layer and ease of suturing of the keratinized gingiva and mucosa. Inappropriate soft-tissue incisions may result in permanent scars and compromise vascularization.

At least one vertical releasing incision should be performed to supplement the crestal and sulcular incisions. An appropriate region is the median labial frenum with its naturally scar-like structure and without large blood vessels crossing the midline. Other appropriate sites for releasing incisions are distal to the maxillary tuberosity or toward the ascending ramus of the mandible, using a 45-degree angled incision. While vertical releasing incisions can also be placed within the marginal gingiva, visible areas should be avoided with scar formation in mind.

Full-thickness flaps should be used in augmentation surgery. These designs offer the benefit of preserving vessels and nerves, and they do not involve scar formation during healing. By maintaining an intact periosteum attached to the flap, vital neighboring structures like the facial nerve and the facial arteries are protected. The flap design should offer both relaxed access to the deficient bone and good overview, including any neighboring structures that the procedure may involve (Figs 3a-d).

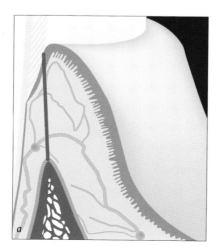 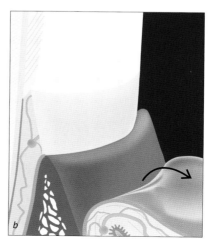

Figs 3a-b Blood supply and incision lines for ridge augmentation/tooth area.

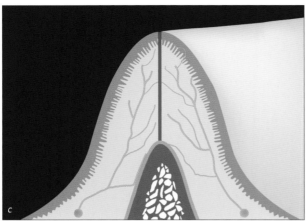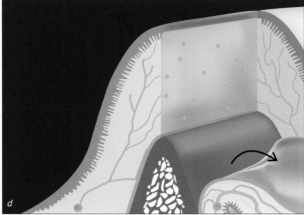

Figs 3 c-d   Blood supply and incision lines for ridge augmentation/edentulous situation.

4.3 Healing of Autologous Bone Block Grafts

Autologous bone blocks can integrate within a relatively short period of 4 to 6 months, turning into new jawbone that can no longer be distinguished from the preexisting native bone in its vicinity (Figs 4a-d). It is a general biological principle that non-vascularized bone grafts will heal by complete osteoclastic degradation and osteoblastic rebuilding. This principle is known as "creeping substitution" (Axhausen 1908; Urist 1965). The first few weeks of bone healing are characterized by woven cancellous bone filling the voids between the autologous bone block and the pristine bone surface (Fig 5). This is followed by a phase of bone tissue growing from the recipient site into the graft. A typical histological formation—i.e. the "cutting cones"—create tunnels from the recipient bone into the grafted bone (Figs 6 and 7). These tunnels are filled by concentric circular layers of lamellar bone. The resultant structure is known as an "osteon" or "Haversian system." This process continues until the grafted bone has been completely replaced by new osteons and become an integral part of the host bone. Several years may pass until remodeling of the grafted bone will be completed.

As shown (Figs 4a-d), a block graft will even heal in the absence of a bone substitute and membrane.

The surgeon should establish intimate contact with the underlying bone on positioning the block into the defect. To this end, the block and the underlying bone should be properly trimmed. Intimate contact will facilitate migration of the cutting cones from the recipient bone into the graft. No bone substitutes or foreign materials are interposed between the block graft and the underlying host bone with this concept. Autologous bone chips should be the only material used to fill a void between the block graft and the recipient bone surface. Importantly, one or more fixation screws must be used to stabilize the block graft.

After 4 to 6 months, the healing process will have progressed sufficiently for the block graft to reach a clinical state of firm attachment to the pristine bone surface. Now the fixation screws can be removed. As noted above, complete remodeling of a grafted bone block may

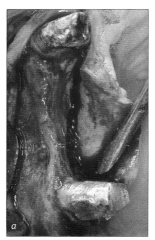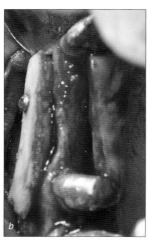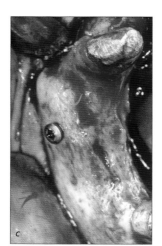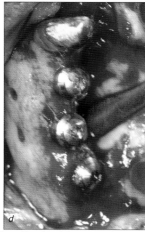

Figs 4a-d   Healing of a block graft in the absence of bone substitute or a membrane. (a) Horizontal defect at baseline. (b) A block harvested from the ramus is secured by one screw without addition of bone chips, bone substitute, or a membrane. (c) After 4 months of healing, the graft is well incorporated. (d) The screw can be removed and the implants placed.

take several years, depending on the patient's age and general skeletal remodeling rate. It is not advisable, however, to wait much longer than 4 to 6 months before placing the dental implants, as the block graft may undergo resorption at the external (periosteal) surface. Various degrees of osteoclastic resorption of the external bone graft surface will take place simultaneously with internal remodeling. The surface resorption will flatten the grafted bone contour and round off sharp edges of the block. Any significant degree of surface resorption is clinically undesirable by potentially involving a loss in graft height

and contour with subsequent recession of the overlying mucosa. Barrier membranes and bone substitutes may help to prevent surface resorption and promote internal remodeling of a grafted bone block (Figs 8a-f) (Cordaro and coworkers 2011b).Once grafted to the alveolar crest, the bone used for augmentation will be completely lost to resorption within a few years unless protected or adequately loaded by occlusal forces via natural teeth or implants. The latter have been shown to protect bone from resorption much like teeth do, presumably because of functional loads being transferred to the jawbone.

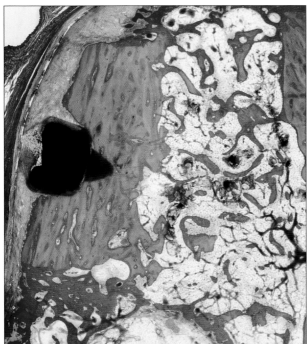

Fig 5   Histological view of a healed bone block. Note the formation of woven bone in contour gaps surrounding the block. The grafted bone itself shows multiple zones of remodeling by new osteons. Also, the surface of the pristine bone has been widely resorbed and remodeled. (Courtesy of Bosshardt and coworkers 2009.)

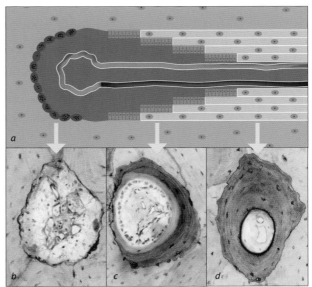

Fig 6   Cutting cones take care of remodeling a free autologous bone graft. Osteoclasts gather around the tip of a vascular loop and will "drill" a tunnel into the graft bone. The tunnel propagates through the graft bone and then gets filled by concentric layers of new lamellar bone. The resultant structure is an osteon, also called a "Haversian system." (Bosshardt DD, Schenk RK. Bone regeneration: biologic basis. In: Buser D, editor. 20 Years of Guided Bone Regeneration in Implant Dentistry. 2nd edn. Chicago, IL: Quintessenz 2009:15–45.)

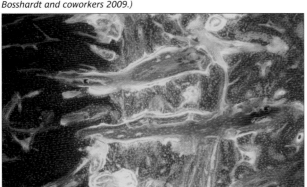

Fig 7   Cutting cones can be seen migrating through a bone graft (sequential intravital fluorochrome staining under UV light).

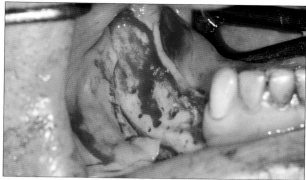

Fig 8a Baseline defect in the posterior mandible. The cortical bone has been perforated with a bur to access the trabecular compartment, and a notch was created.

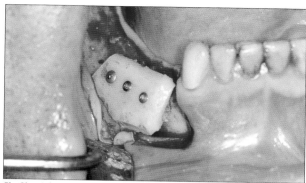

Fig 8b A bone block from the external oblique ridge is secured in the notch with three titanium positioning screws. The graft overlaps the crest of the ridge (shell technique) to compensate for the vertical component of the 3/4 defect.

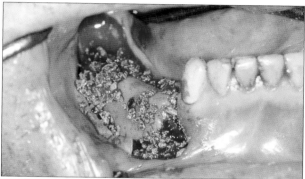

Fig 8c A mixed particulate graft (75% demineralized bone matrix and 25% autologous bone chips) fills the void behind the bone block and around the block to level out the contour.

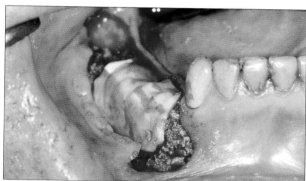

Fig 8d A resorbable collagen membrane is placed over the graft.

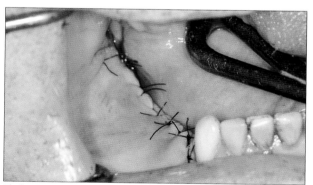

Fig 8e Wound closure with interrupted sutures.

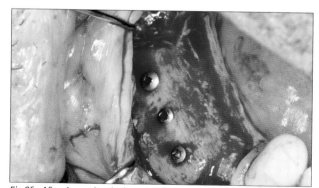

Fig 8f After 4 months, the bone block is incorporated, along with the surrounding particulated material, in new bone. After removing the titanium screws, the stage is set for implant placement. The bone block will have another 3 to 4 months for integration and remodeling while the implants are undergoing osseointegration.

4.4 Harvesting Autologous Bone from Intraoral Sites

Bone may be harvested from several intraoral sites, most commonly in the mandible from the buccal cortical plate of the horizontal ramus or the symphysial (chin) area (Clavero and Lundgren 2003). The maxillary tuberosity area and the zygomaticoalveolar crest are also used. Limited amounts of bone chips can also be harvested locally with bone scrapers from the surgical implant site, eliminating the need for a second surgical wound. Most patients will experience less discomfort from intraoral than extraoral donor sites, as recently demonstrated in a controlled study comparing effects of extra versus intraoral donor sites on OHRQOL-HRQOL (oral-health-related and health-related quality of life) outcomes (Reissmann and coworkers 2013).

4.4.1 Harvesting Bone from the Mandibular Ramus

Bone from the mandibular ramus and angle as donor site is usually harvested by elevating only the outer cortical plate, the surgical rationale being that confining the procedure to the cortical portion of the mandible will eliminate the risk of injury to the mandibular canal or any teeth located within the cancellous portion of the mandible almost completely (Nkenke and coworkers 2001; Raghoebar and coworkers 2001).

If the mandibular molars are present, two alternative incision lines can be used to access the area: either a marginal incision with a short oblique releasing incision toward the ascending ramus, or an incision directly over the external oblique ridge within the alveolar mucosa. The first variant (i.e. the marginal incision) is usually started in the gingival sulcus of the first molar and is then extended in an oblique direction distally and buccally in the retromolar area. There is no need for an anterior releasing incision (Fig 9).

A less preferable variant is a paramarginal incision within the alveolar mucosa, starting at least 3 mm buccal from the mucogingival junction of the first molar, its course parallel to the line connecting the buccal surfaces of the lower cuspid and premolar toward the coronoid process (Figs 10 and 12).

If grafting is planned in the posterior mandible and the molars there are missing, the same flap is used for both the donor and the recipient site. The procedure is started by performing sulcular incisions at the residual teeth (premolars or canines) and extending them distally at the crest of the ridge, splitting the keratinized tissue in two. Then the incision line is angled (45°) and extended buccally toward the ascending ramus in the third-molar region (Figs 11 and 13).

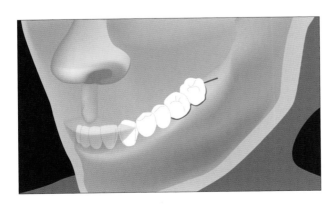

Fig 9   *A marginal incision along the distal teeth with an oblique releasing incision allows the region of the mandibular angle and ramus to be broadly exposed for bone harvesting. Vascularization to the flap is preserved, and scar formation will be minimal.*

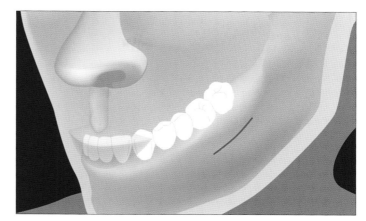

Fig 10   Paramarginal incision.

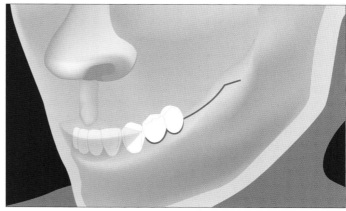

Fig 11   Incision line in a partially edentulous situation.

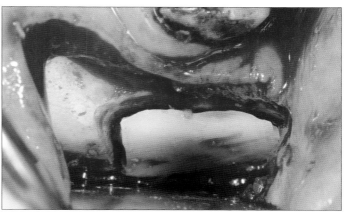

Fig 12   Paramarginal incision to access the external portion of the mandibular angle and ramus, performed directly superior to the external oblique ridge (linea obliqua externa) at least 3 mm buccal to the mucogingival junction. On the lingual side of the incision, a wide soft-tissue pedicle is retained to facilitate subsequent closure of the wound. This image displays the situation with the osteotomies already performed.

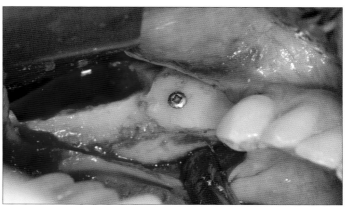

Fig 13   Incision line to harvest bone from the ramus for grafting in the posterior mandible if the molars are missing. Harvesting and grafting can be performed through the same flap.

It is essential for a safe and effective surgical procedure to elevate a clean full-thickness flap. Bone management under an intact periosteal layer buccal to the lateral portion of the mandible will ensure a lower risk to vessels and nerves (i.e. injury to the facial artery or the marginal mandibular branch of the facial nerve).

Raising a flap with an intact periosteal layer may be a challenge if the incision is performed within the alveolar mucosa. Access should be established with a deep incision line closely approaching the bone directly buccal to the molars and superior to the external oblique ridge. A single accurate cut is required to incise the periosteum, elevating it medially to expose the bone adjacent to the molars. This thin flap will be very useful with a view to achieving wound closure in layers after harvesting.

Subperiosteal preparation of the buccal angle and ramus portion should be carried out next (Figs 14a-p). The design of this flap will—regardless of the selected incision—depend on the amount of bone needed. As only 10–25 mm of cortical height are normally harvested from this area, the inferior border of the mandible is not usually involved. In preparing the outer portion of the mandible, the soft tissues should be retracted to view the base of the coronoid process. This marks the end of soft-tissue preparation, as the bony structure is now widely exposed.

The ensuing bone surgery is usually initiated by performing two bone cuts into the ramus on its lateral aspect, starting at the level of the external oblique ridge and proceeding obliquely toward the mandibular angle (Fig 14g). These parallel osteotomies establish the length and height of the graft. They only involve the cor-

tical aspect of the mandible and are stopped on the first sign of bleeding from marrow bone. The width of the graft will depend on the width of the cortical bone.

Commencement of bleeding indicates that drilling has reached the cancellous bone at the osteotomy site. A third osteotomy is performed to connect the former two on the lateral and superior aspects of the retromolar region, parallel and medial to the external oblique ridge. This osteotomy is usually not carried out until the former two have been completed, as the surgeon cannot evaluate the exact width of the cortical plate before that point.

A straight handpiece with thin osteotomy burs (Lindemann) is used to perform the osteotomies. Alternatively, a piezoelectric device may be applied.

It may be helpful to perform a bone cut into the apical cortical plate with a round medium-sized bur, a protected circular saw, or a piezoelectric angled handpiece to define the height of the cortical bone block and to ensure controlled fracture of the harvested bone. A bone trap can be used to collect particles. Subsequently, the rest of the apical cortical plate may be fractured, without encroaching on the cancellous component, with a periosteal elevator.

After harvesting a flat block of cortical bone, whose dimensions may vary, the cancellous compartment of the mandible will be clearly visible. In rare cases, the intact alveolar nerve will be apparent too. A collagen sponge or similar biomaterial may be packed to the site and antibiotics added. The block may be used as a single piece or divided into segments.

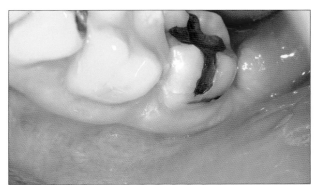

Fig 14a   Retromolar area. Mandibular block anesthesia has been performed.

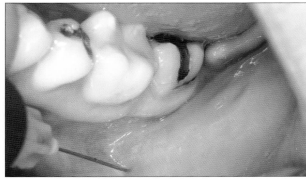

Fig 14b   Infiltration with local anesthesia for pain control in the region of the masseter muscle.

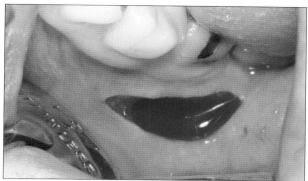

Fig 14c   Incision line just superficial to the external oblique ridge (linea obliqua externa).

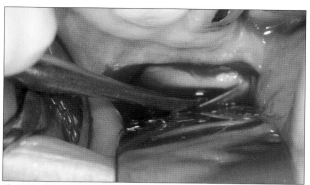

Fig 14d   Subperiosteal dissection of the buccal portion of the horizontal mandibular ramus.

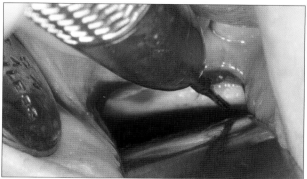

Fig 14e   A straight handpiece is used for the osteotomies. The first two parallel osteotomies are performed into the cortical plate, starting at the external oblique ridge and continuing toward the inferior border of the mandible.

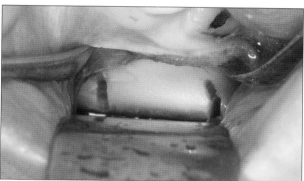

Fig 14f   The osteotomy remains limited to cortical bone. Bleeding defines the point at which cortical turns into cancellous bone (location of the mandibular neurovascular bundle).

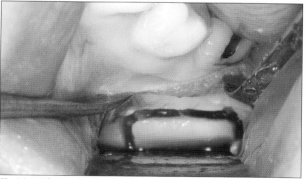

Fig 14g   After evaluating the thickness of the buccal cortical plate, the sagittal upper osteotomy is designed and completed.

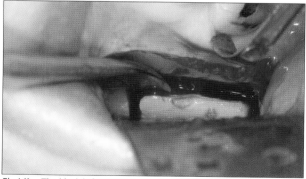

Fig 14h   The block is fractured by blunt application of a periosteal elevator.

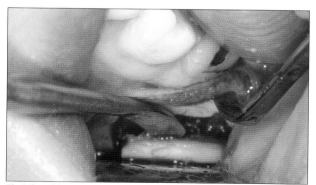

Fig 14i   Initial graft mobilization.

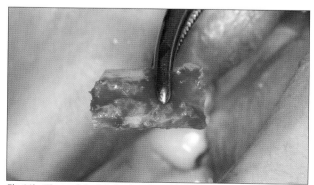

Fig 14j   The graft is dislodged and used in its current block form or after abrasive treatment.

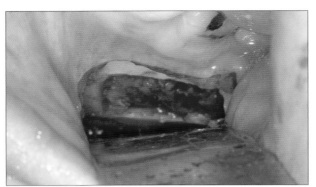

Fig 14k   Donor site immediately after block harvesting.

Also, the block may be ground in a bone mill, entirely or in part, to be used as a particulate graft (Fig 15). Wound closure should be completed with care. If the soft-tissue incision has been performed within the alveolar mucosa, the wound should be closed in layers, including a first suture line with resorbable stitches that includes the periosteum and muscles and a second suture line that closes the mucosal layer. If a marginal incision was used, single stitches at the level of the papillae and the distal portion of the incision are the way to go.

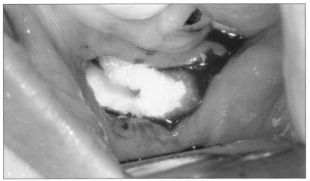

Fig 14l   A collagen sponge is placed in the wound to prepare for suturing.

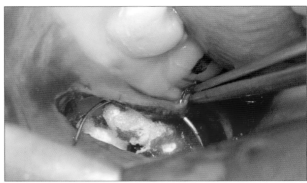

Fig 14m   The wound needs to be sutured in layers, involving the muscle and the periosteal layer on the medial part of the wound.

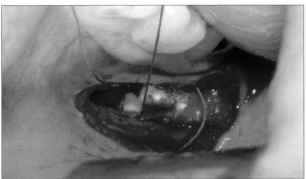

Fig 14n   Buccal muscle layer with the suture, just before tying the knot.

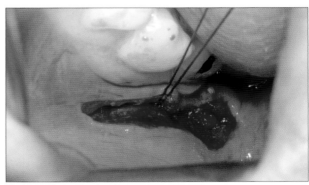

Fig 14o   Closing the deep layer.

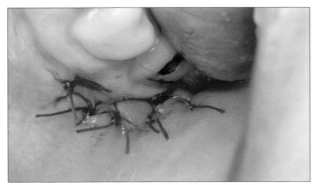

Fig 14p   Closing the mucosal layer with interrupted sutures.

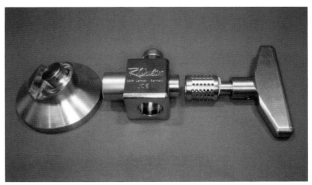

Fig 15   Bone mill.

4.4.2 Bone Harvesting from the Anterior Mandible (Chin)

Two factors are essential to safe and effective bone harvesting from the chin: the mental foramina and nerves must be protected, and effective wound closure needs to be ensured with the insertions of the mentalis muscles preserved. The way to accomplish this is by using a precise incision design and carefully exposing the chin area.

Two incision lines may be used: either a horizontal incision deep in the vestibule, cutting through the mentalis muscles, or a long vertical midline incision going directly to the bone.

Soft-tissue preparation for the first of these two (horizontal) approaches is started by performing a horizontal incision from cuspid to cuspid in the buccal vestibule approximately 10 mm away from the mucogingival junction. Subsequently, the incision is advanced deeper within the muscle layer in an oblique posterior direction toward the periosteum, such that a wide band of tissue is left pedicled to the mandible at the coronal level, which will permit wound closure in layers and readaptation of the mentalis muscle to prevent chin ptosis.

Then the periosteum is elevated toward the inferior border, resulting in exposure of the anterior mandible. If necessary, the dissection may be extended toward the distal (without broadening the mucosal incision) to bilaterally expose the mental foramina. At this point, it is mandatory for the surgeon to assess the position of anatomical limitations before proceeding. Landmarks needed to outline the area in which the osteotomy will be performed include the positions of the anterior tooth apices, the mental foramina, and the inferior border of the mandible. A safety margin of at least 5 mm from the mental foramina and the mandibular anterior tooth apices should be respected.

Harvesting deep blocks (including cancellous bone) clearly involves a high risk of damaging the incisive branch of the inferior alveolar nerve. It is for this reason that sensitivity loss of the mandibular incisors is frequently seen after bone harvesting from the chin. While this loss is temporary in the vast majority of patients, some may not respond to pulp sensitivity testing for several years. Postoperative problems with lip sensory function is avoided by taking the surgical approach here described.

Bone from the chin is usually harvested with trephine burs of various diameters (7–12 mm) in a handpiece. Depending on the required dimensions of the graft, bony cylinders of different diameters and depths are created (Fig 16h). Copious irrigation with sterile saline is mandatory, as trephine burs tend to produce heat. A range of different burs but also saws or piezoelectric devices may be used to create blocks of various shapes and sizes.

For rectangular blocks, the mandibular ramus offers a lower complication rate and is therefore the donor site of choice. The chin remains the donor site of choice for corticocancellous blocks or grafts thicker than 4 mm. Note that the use of a curette or forceps in harvesting cancellous bone may increase the risk of damaging vascular supply to the mandibular anterior teeth.

As noted above, great care must be taken when applying the trephines to leave at least 5 mm of intact bone underneath the mandibular roots. Up to four cylinders may be prepared, and an ample volume of bone can be harvested. A straight elevator is normally used to separate the blocks from the mandible once the osteotomy with burs or piezosurgical devices has been accomplished, usually followed by filling the defect with a collagen sponge or a similar resorbable material to which an antibiotic powder or solution may be added.

Any need for particulate grafts (e.g. in procedures of sinus floor augmentation) may then be covered by partial or complete milling of the bone blocks or cylinders with the aid of a bone mill (see Fig 15).

The next step is to achieve layered wound closure. It is vital to suture the periosteal and muscle layers before suturing the mucosal layer, avoiding the complication of lowerlip and chin ptosis and its potential consequence of increased lower-incisor visibility. Resorbable inverted sutures are used to close the deeper periosteal and muscle layers, such that the knot is displaced within the tissues. Once the muscle layer has been closed, multiple single or continuous sutures are used to close the mucosal layer. To reduce postoperative swelling and promote safe healing of the mentalis muscle, an external compressive dressing should be applied with adhesive tape from ear to ear and will normally be removed a few days later (Figs 16a-o) (Chaushu and coworkers 2001).

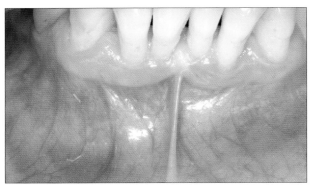

Fig 16a   Case illustrating the horizontal incision approach to harvesting bone from the symphysial (chin) region of the mandible. Clinical view of the anterior mandible prior to local anesthetic infiltration.

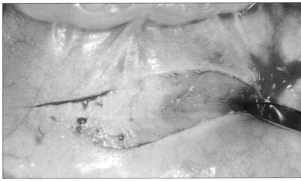

Fig 16b   A superficial horizontal incision is performed, respecting a minimum distance from the mucogingival line of 3 mm.

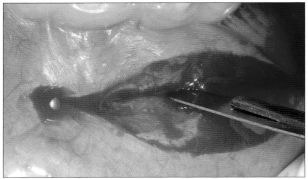

Fig 16c   The incision is then deepened in an oblique posterior direction toward the periosteal layer, such that contact with the bone is made apical to the root apices of the lower incisors.

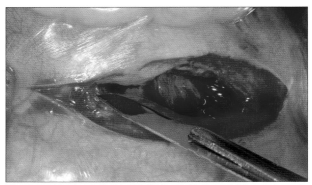

Fig 16d   A broad muscle layer is left attached to the cranial wound margin.

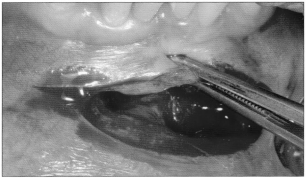

Fig 16e   The cranial flap will allow for layered suturing once bone harvesting has been completed.

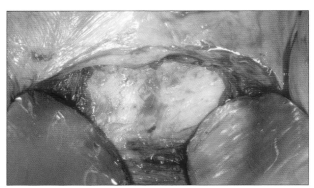

Fig 16f   Broad exposure of the chin area.

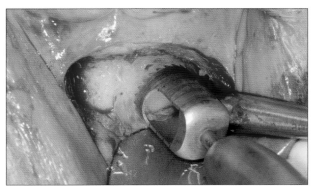

Fig 16g   Trephine burs of varying diameters may be used to design the osteotomies for bone harvesting.

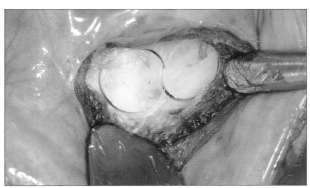

Fig 16h   Round cylinders ready to be harvested.

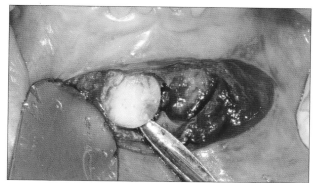

Fig 16i   Removal of the bone block using a straight elevator.

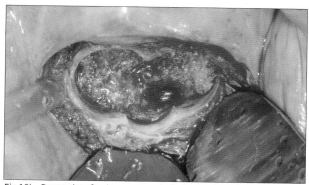

Fig 16j   Donor site after bone removal, displaying the residual component of cancellous bone.

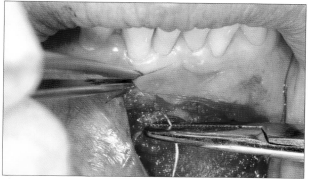

Fig 16k   A layered approach to suturing is taken, starting with the muscle layer.

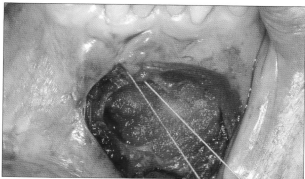

Fig 16l   The bone defect has been filled with a collagen sponge after harvesting. A resorbable material is used to pass the first suture through the muscle layer of the cranial flap, taking an inverted direction.

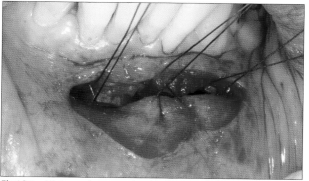

Fig 16m   All deep sutures are placed before completing the knots.

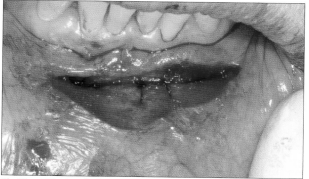

Fig 16n   This view displays the sutured muscle layer.

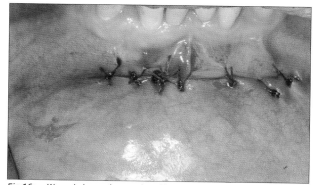

Fig 16o   Wound closure is completed by adding interrupted sutures at the mucosal level.

4.5 Harvesting of Autologous Bone from Extraoral Sites

Bone from extraoral sites may be indicated to meet graft volume requirements, to offer better resistance to resorption, or to ensure safer and faster healing than with grafts that could be harvested from intraoral sites.

4.5.1 Iliac Bone Grafts

Iliac bone is usually a source of adequately voluminous and sizable grafts to treat even large bone defects up to hemi-mandibles following resections (Figs 17a-r). Material harvested in this way offers superior cell density and regenerative capacity in comparison with intraoral bone blocks (Springer and coworkers 2004). The preferred donor site for more extensive bone requirements is the inner table of the iliac wing. Harvesting is usually performed under general anesthesia. There is no need for an extended skin incision, since the surgical access can be shifted back and forth over the donor region. All it takes is a short skin incision, which will result in a minor scar. It is advisable to perform the incision parallel and a little cranial to the palpable crest in the direction of the relaxed skin-tension lines. Care must be taken to spare the cutaneous femoral lateral nerve, which runs from the inside of the iliac wing around the anterior iliac spine. To minimize postoperative pain, the incisions should not pass through the abdominal and gluteal muscles; they should be placed in the aponeurosis between these muscles on top of the crest, keeping the gluteal muscles firmly attached.

The rounded contour of the compact bone at the inner aspect of the anterior iliac crest can preferably be used to rebuild a well-rounded alveolar crest contour. Larger pieces featuring a rounded contour for a complete maxillary onlay graft can also be obtained from the outer posterior aspect of the anterior crest (Lundgren and Sennerby 2008). Advanced computer-aided methods can be used to optimize the shape of iliac-bone pieces such that they will accurately fit into the defect. Iliac anatomy is relatively constant, however, such that preoperative imaging is often not required in the hands of experienced

surgeons. An oscillating saw is the preferred tool for harvesting, as chisels lead to uncontrolled cracks that may later turn into fractures. Corticocancellous blocks are harvested monocortically from the inside of the iliac wing for applications of implant dentistry, keeping the crest and the external plate with their muscle attachments intact. After bleeding has been stopped with bone wax and placing a drain without suction, the wound is finally closed in three layers.

A minimally invasive approach can be taken to harvest small amounts of cancellous bone from the iliac site by the use of trephines, with a stab incision through the skin. Local anesthesia will be sufficient in this situation. While it is both easier and meets with better patient acceptance to harvest bone from the posterior from the anterior iliac crest, this involves a time-consuming intraoperative manipulation of turning the patient. Harvesting from the posterior crest is accomplished via a skin incision directly over the palpable medial part of the posterior iliac crest; access is difficult to establish in overweight patients.

Postoperatively, a bupivacaine depot injection and a supporting elastic bandage are recommended for pain relief. The patient will use forearm crutches for several days and, while permitted to load his or her limbs and to move freely, should not allow the loading to reach pain level. Typical complications include pain, gait disturbance, and sensory problems in the lateral thigh area. Osteoporotic patients may experience iliac-wing fractures, most of which will be conservatively treated. Although severe complications like abdominal perforations or infections are rare, iliac-bone grafts should be harvested by surgeons capable of managing such events. Due to its low complication rate, the anterior iliac crest is the most preferred and recommended extraoral source of bone. A prospective study of 235 iliac-bone procedures did not reveal any severe complications, and the level of postoperative pain and complications was low and acceptable (Barone and coworkers 2011).

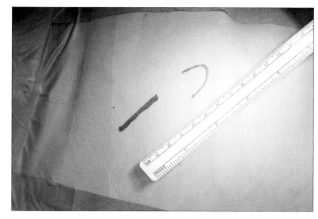

Fig 17a   Clinical case of iliac-bone harvesting: right lateral abdominal area, leg on the right, chest toward the left. The skin had been washed with a disinfectant iodine solution and the area isolated with adhesive dressings to create a sterile surgical field. The semicircular mark indicates the palpable anterior iliac spine. Care must be taken to avoid this area, since this is where the lateral femoral nerve runs from the abdominal side. The bold straight mark is 3 cm long and was drawn to show the skin incision line slightly cranial to the iliac crest. This incision should not be placed directly over the crest, since this is where the patient will wear a waistband or a belt.

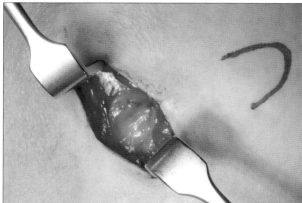

Fig 17b   The skin incision is followed by dissecting the underlying fat and meticulous hemostasis.

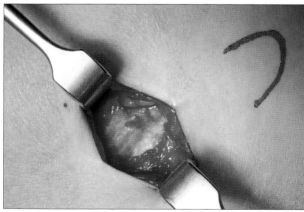

Fig 17c   At this point, the dissection has reached the lateral oblique striated abdominal muscle (above) and the white aponeurosis of the insertion of the gluteal muscle on top of the anterior iliac crest. The aponeurosis is carefully cut in the middle, without cutting into the abdominal muscle and not detaching the muscular insertion from the lateral side of the crest.

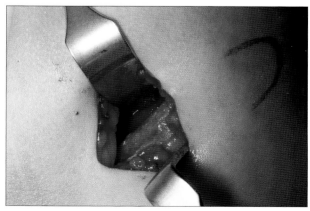

Fig 17d   The periosteum is stripped off the inner iliac table to expose the bone crest. A large bone surface can be approached through just a little skin opening by moving the short (3 cm) incision up and down the crest, minimizing trauma.

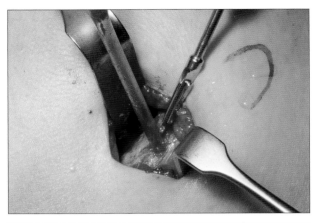

Fig 17e   An oscillating saw is used to split the crest longitudinally under copious irrigation with saline.

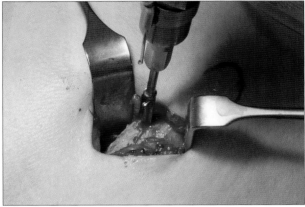

Fig 17f   A transverse cut is performed with the oscillating saw 2 cm behind the anterior iliac spine. Then the soft tissues are moved backward with the retractor to perform another transverse bone cut at the posterior extension of the block graft. The corticotomy is then completed via a final cut performed on the inner table parallel to the crestal cut.

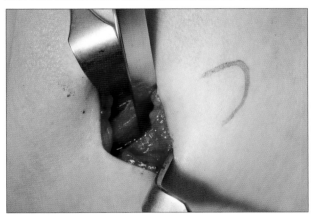

Fig 17g   Using a straight-blade osteotome, the monocortical bone block graft is detached from the adhesions of the cancellous bone underneath. The instrument should be handled very gently to avoid inducing cracks and fractures, notably in osteoporotic patients. Normally the cancellous bone is rather soft and amenable to cutting without much force.

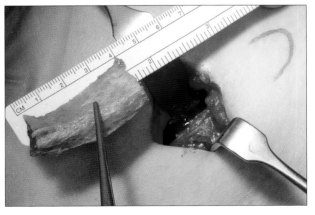

Fig 17h   Harvesting of a monocortical corticocancellous block. By moving the soft tissues back and forth, it becomes possible to harvest a graft much larger than the soft-tissue incision. Care has been taken to protect all relevant muscle structures and insertions to minimize postoperative pain.

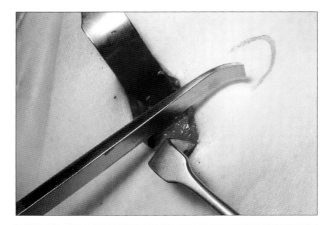

Fig 17i   Several vertical bone cuts are made with the oscillating saw in the inner table to harvest strips of monocortical bone. A special osteotome featuring a curved blade (according to Obwegeser) is used to detach these strips in the depth of the inner iliac table.

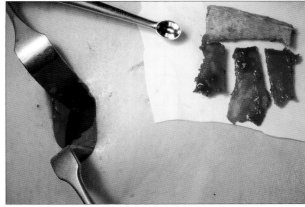

Fig 17j   These strips of monocortical bone have been harvested from the inner iliac table. A large curette is used to collect more cancellous bone.

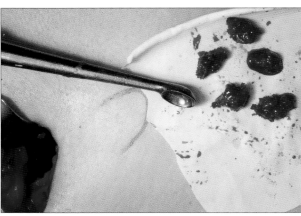

Fig 17k   Cancellous bone which has been additionally harvested with a curette.

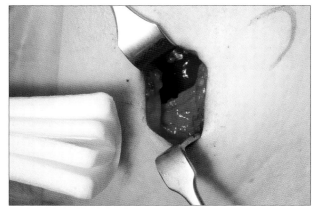

Fig 17l   Hemostasis and defect filling is achieved with a large oversized and folded piece of collagen fleece (Resorba, Nürnberg, Germany), which shrinks inside the wound, soaks blood, and triggers clotting. Severe bleeding may indicate the additional use of bone wax. Also, a Redon drain without suction can be placed in severe cases of bleeding.

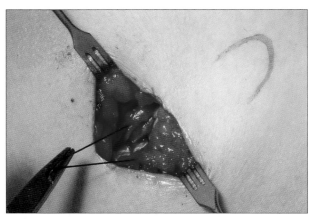

Fig 17m   The first step toward wound closure is to readapt the white aponeurosis in a mechanically stable fashion using three Vicryl (Ethicon, Norderstedt, Germany) size-1 threads. The next layer—the subcutaneous fat—is closed with Vicryl 3-0.

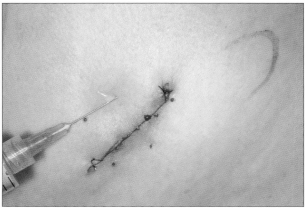

Fig 17n   The skin is closed with a continuous intradermal 4-0 monofilament polyamide thread. The surrounding soft tissues are infiltrated by 10 ml of bupivacaine 0.5% solution with adrenaline.

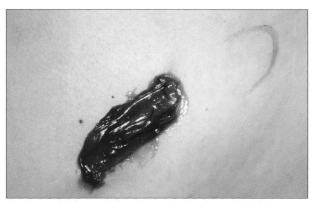

Fig 17o   A disinfectant iodine ointment is placed over the incision.

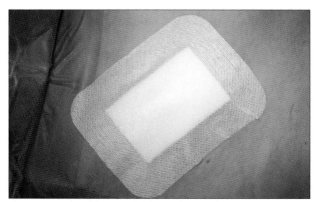

Fig 17p   Dressing of the wound with a small piece of sterile adhesive plaster.

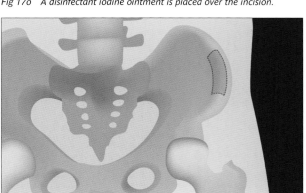

Fig 17q   Schematic drawing of donor site.

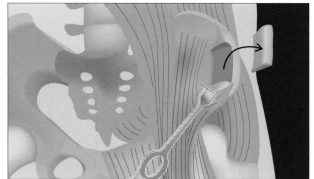

Fig 17r   Schematic of the muscle insertion and its relevance for the harvesting procedure.

4.5.2 Calvarial Bone

Cortical bone from the skull is one of the structures offering the highest mineral densities in the human body—higher than those of cortical bone from other extraoral sites and even higher than the mineral density of mandibular bone. Skull bone is therefore considered highly resistant to resorption, even outperforming mandibular cortical bone in this respect (Chiapasco and coworkers 2013), and offers relatively predictable healing in intraoral recipient sites. It can be harvested under local anesthesia, though general anesthesia is used more commonly due to the surgery-related bone concussion and noise. It is harvested from the parietal bone, bilateral to the sagittal suture, where the skull has its greatest thickness and the inner table is separated from the outer table by a defined diploic layer (Figs 18 a-d).

A longitudinal incision 10 cm in length is performed 5 cm laterally parallel to the sagittal suture, through the skin, the epicranial muscle, and the galea aponeuratica. As the scalp is rich in blood vessels, Raney clips are placed on the skin margins to control bleeding. A wound spreader is used. After the grafts have been outlined with a bur, wide and flat access osteotomies 1 cm in width are created around the block grafts with a round bur or a piezosurgical device. A substantial amount of bone needs to be removed to offer access for a flat chisel to split the outer calvarian table from the inner table; the latter is left intact. An alternative tool for splitting would be to use an oscillating saw. Blocks thus obtained are usually 4–5 mm thick and include cancellous bone from the diploe. Throughout the osteotomies, a bone trap should be used to collect chips. Some authors have proposed to also harvest pieces of pericranium for use as natural collagen membranes (Chiapasco and coworkers 2013). Bleeding from the diploic veins is stopped with bone wax. Resorbable 1-0 sutures are used in the galea and subcutaneously for wound closure, then closing the skin with a 3-0 monofilament polyamide suture. A suction drain is placed under the galea.

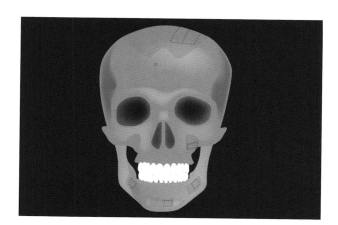

Fig 18a   Size and amount of bone grafts that can be harvested from intra- and extraoral donor sites of the calvarium.

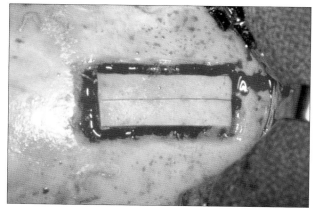

Fig 18b   Harvesting of a calvarial bone graft from the outer parietal table. Two rectangular strips of bone are cut with an oscillating saw. Cortical bone around the grafts is removed with a round bur to create access for flat osteotome chisels to split the diploic layer. Care is taken not to fracture the inner calvarial table.

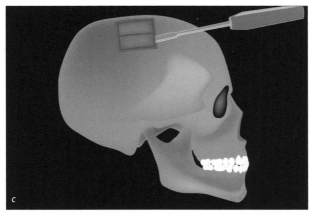

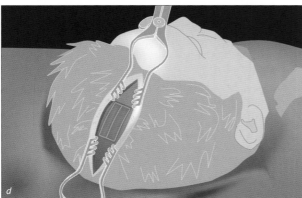

Fig18c-d   The graft is removed by dividing the bone into several segments (depending on the bone quantity required for grafting), which are then removed one by one. Chisels are used to dislodge the graft from the inner table.

Donor site morbidity is generally low if bone grafts from the skull are properly harvested, and the donor defects will be replenished with new bone quickly. Nevertheless, calvarial grafting has a potential of causing severe complications, including lifethreatening events of intracerebral hemorrhage, skull fracture, intracranial penetration. Major complications have been reported to occur with a relatively high incidence of 19.2% (Scheerlinck and coworkers 2013). Bone harvesting from the skull is not a routine procedure in oral surgery and should be performed exclusively by maxillofacial surgeons who are capable of managing potential complications. An advantage of this site is that the scar remains masked by hair (unless the patient is bald).

4.5.3   Other Extraoral Sites

In addition to the iliac crest and skull, a few other extraoral sites have been used to harvest bone for grafting. While example like the ribs or long bones are generally not recommended for use in implant dentistry, the tibial head has gained some popularity as a donor site for cancellous bone. Unlike iliac and intraoral harvesting, however, this approach cannot be considered a routine procedure in oral surgery due to the reduced volume and low mineral density of the cancellous bone available from the tibial head (Engelstad and Morse 2010). In addition, the limbs offer a reduced healing potential in case of infectious complications.

4.6 Bone Quality and Quantity

The iliac crest is an ample source of autologous bone that will suffice even for major reconstructions. Its cancellous part has often been termed the "gold standard" for bone grafts, due to its high content of osteogenic cells offering an excellent healing capacity. Also, these grafts are suitable for a wide range of applications in implant dentistry. Corticancellous grafts from the internal side of the anterior crest are relatively soft in structure, comparable to type D3/D4 bone according to the Misch classification (Misch 1989). Given its abundance of living bone cells, grafts from the iliac crest will heal more quickly than grafts from intraoral donor sites. At the same time, however, they will also resorb at a faster rate than cortical bone blocks harvested from the oral cavity, which is compounded by the potentially unpredictable nature of this resorption notably in onlay grafts. Even proper loading by dental implants may not prevent continued resorption of these grafts for up to several years (Wiltfang and coworkers 2012).

Skull bone is a matrix consisting purely of compact bone with a very high mineral density. It is therefore highly resistant to uncontrolled resorption and has often been used in implant dentistry for this reason, especially in onlay grafting of resorbed edentulous ridges. Cortical bone is considered to harbor fewer stem cells but more growth factors and bone-morphogenetic proteins (BMP) stored in the bone matrix than cancellous bone.

High mineral density is also offered by intraoral bone grafts from the mandible. Bone harvested from the ramus or chin will differ in quality. Harvesting from the ramus must remain confined to cortical bone as a function of surgical technique and the presence of the alveolar nerve and root tips. Of course, this cortical bone can be milled and used for inlay grafting as in sinus surgery. Unlike the ramus, the chin is a viable source for corticocancellous blocks. As stated previously, this donor site should be selected whenever there is a need for an intraorally trephined and large corticocancellous graft. It should be noted that only part of a chin block can be milled, leaving the cortical portion intact for use as a screwed block graft for horizontal or vertical augmentation.

Considerable amounts of grafting material can be harvested from the mandible. They have been used to accomplish bilateral cases of sinus floor elevation (Cordaro and coworkers 2011b) and full-arch maxillary reconstructions of complete edentulism (Cordaro and coworkers 2012a; Schwartz-Arad and Lewin 2005).

4.7 Biomaterials: Selection of Bone Substitutes and Membranes

The natural matrix for all bone healing is the fibrin of the blood clot. Bone chips and grafts are capable of accelerating the healing process, as autologous bone functions as a scaffold for new bone formation. They are also known to contribute osteogenic stem cells and growth and differentiation factors that chemically bind to proteins in the autologous bone matrix. One group of these growth factors—the bone-morphogenetic proteins (BMPs)—will induce precursor cells to differentiate into bone forming cells. Bone precursor cells are capable of migrating over the bone surface and detaching growth factors through the action of specific enzymes. It is therefore beneficial to make the growth factors accessible to the cells by subjecting the bone graft to grinding, chipping, or milling.

Unlike the pure blood clot, most bone substitutes will mechanically impede early neoangiogenesis and bone regeneration. To allow vascular ingrowth and cell migration into the augmented volume, they should not be packed too densely. Also, much like particulated grafts, which by their physical nature usually include open interconnective spaces between the particles, bone substitutes should contain interconnective pores as well. A pore size greater than 300 µm is biologically ideal for vascular ingrowth and subsequent ossification (Karageorgiou and Kaplan 2005). Furthermore, bone substitutes are used as a passive filler to support the membrane and to define the contour of the graft. Clinicians should keep in mind that every bone substitute is a foreign body that should never elicit an immune response by antigenicity. Sterile inflammation may occur by small foreign particles and dust stimulating a macrophage-mediated immune response (Anderson and coworkers 2008).

Deproteinized bovine bone matrix (DBBM) is a well-documented bone substitute offering a low substitution rate for intraoral grafting. A suitable alternative for patients who prefer synthetic materials is biphasic hydroxyapatite plus tricalcium phosphate (Straumann Bone Ceramic®; Straumann, Basel, Switzerland). Both materials have been demonstrated to be osteoconductive (Jensen and coworkers 2007). In other words, they are known promote a certain extent of slow appositional bone growth from the bony walls into the defect. This appositional growth depends on the growth of new blood vessels between the particles. In the alveolar crest, it spontaneously stops at a distance of few millimeters above the defect bone wall. The more distant particles heal within fibrous tissue to form a scar. A barrier membrane can be used to increase the distance of vascular ingrowth into a bone graft and subsequent ossification. It should be noted that the bone substitute materials just mentioned are not osteoinductive. In other words, they do not induce bone formation via differentiation of mesenchymal stem cells by BMP, which implies that osteoinductivity does not depend on a bony site but may also take the form of ectopic ossification. Osteoinductive properties may be introduced to the graft by mixing the bone substitute particles with autologous bone chips, which is why larger defects should be managed with mixed grafts rather than with bone substitute alone.

In a number of countries, allogeneic bone grafts derived from cadavers have gained some popularity to reduce the need for autologous bone harvesting. The included residual bioactivity of BMP depends on the aggressiveness of the methods used to disinfect these products, which includes simple freezing, chemically cleaned allogeneic bone, or bone that has been sterilized with high doses of gamma radiation. Also, the risk of disease transmission varies with the sterilization techniques employed. HIV transmission via bank bone has been reported to occur (Schratt and coworkers 1996; Simonds 1993). Another problem is contamination with sporeforming bacteria that resist disinfection (Simonpieri and coworkers 2009), and immunogenic effects of allografts vary with the aforementioned processing techniques as well.

A well-documented type of resorbable barrier membrane is the porcine, non-crosslinked, natural collagen membrane. This hydrophilic material integrates well with the fibrin from the blood clot in the wound, which will normally facilitate clinical handling by not requiring additional fixation by nails or pins. Compared to expanded polytetrafluoroethylene (e-PTFE) membranes, there is a lower tendency for soft-tissue dehiscence and intraoral membrane exposure (Jensen and Terheyden 2009). Disadvantages of resorbable collagen membranes include their relatively fast resorption within 4 to 8 weeks and lack of stiffness requiring the use of filler materials underneath to support the augmentative contour.

A human study has shown that chemical crosslinking of the collagen in the membrane for a more durable barrier function is clinically associated with an increased rate of intraoral membrane exposure (Becker and coworkers 2009). A relatively recent development has been to make resorbable membranes from polyethylene glycol (PEG). This material offers a soft consistency when applied, then turn hard and stiff at the augmentation site. A first study has yielded promising results (Ramel and coworkers 2012; Jung and coworkers 2009).

The most extensively documented type of non-resorbable barrier membrane is made from expanded polytetrafluoroethylene (e-PTFE). Although these membranes perform excellently in terms of augmentative outcomes, they are rather technique sensitive and have often been reported to involve high rates of premature membrane exposure (Chiapasco and coworkers 2006b).

To summarize, the objectives of functional longevity and biocompatibility do not seem to be readily reconcilable in barrier membranes. A stable membrane does not integrate well with tissues but tends to involve gaps prone to bacterial colonization and soft-tissue dehiscence in intraoral environments. Conversely, collagen membranes offering high biocompatibility are presumably not identified as foreign by the body, getting quickly degraded by the continuous proteolytic activity that is part of the natural turnover of connective tissue.

4.8 Mixed Bone Grafts

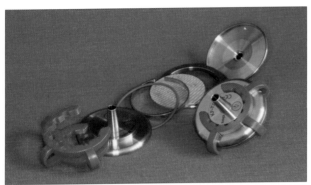

Fig 19 Reusable bone trap for use inside the surgical suction device (Schlumbohm, Pinneberg, Germany)

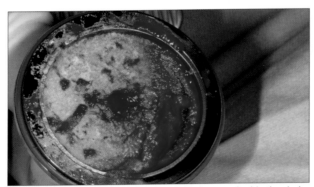

Fig 20 Bone particles after an osteotomy, harvested with the device shown in Fig 16g. To minimize bacterial contamination of the material, the filter should be used during the osteotomy exclusively.

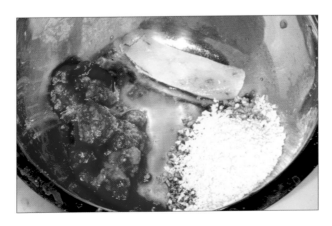

In clinical practice, the properties of autologous bone and bone substitutes are frequently combined for synergy, which is achieved either by layering the materials or by mixing them in particulated form. Particulated intraoral bone is readily available just by using a bone trap, which is a filter inside the surgical suction device (Figs 19 and 20). The rationale of layering grafts is to place the autologous particles, being the more active part, closer to the implant, while the substitute particles are placed closer to the periphery of the defect where they create a smooth outer contour of the bony regenerate for the overlying soft tissues (Buser and coworkers 2008).

Replacing part of an autologous graft volume with a bone substitute can also serve as a means to reduce the surgical burden imposed on a patient by implant dentistry. Nowadays a wide spectrum of implant-related defects can be treated by combining intraoral bone with a bone substitute. There is less of a need for extraoral bone harvesting than there used to be.

What remains unclear even today is the optimal ratio of bone substitute to autologous bone chips in mixed grafts. Animal studies of sinus floor grafting revealed higher bone-to-implant contact rates with mixed grafts than with bone substitutes by themselves, regardless of whether the bone graft had been harvested from the iliac crest or the mandible. Higher shares of autologous bone in the mix were found to increasingly expedite healing (Jensen and coworkers 2013) and higher shares of bone substitute to increasingly reduce shrinkage (Jensen and coworkers 2012) (Fig 21). Bone healing and graft shrinkage turned out to be opposing aims in these animal experiments, a compromise being 25% – 50% of autologous bone in particulated mixed grafts.

Fig 21 Typical grafting materials for bone augmentation. The cortical bone block was harvested from the external oblique ridge with a Lindemann bur. It was 22 × 8 mm in area and consisted purely of cortical bone. The bone chips were collected in the filter as the osteotomy for the block was being performed. Round burs were used to smooth the edges of the defect. An equal amount of deproteinized bovine bone material (DBBM), which is shown in the lower right portion of the dish, was soaked with autologous blood drawn from the vein and was mixed with the autologous chips to form a 50/50 mixed bone graft.

4.9 Fixation of Block Grafts Using Plates and Screws

Block grafts provide volume, mechanical structure, and stability. Those consisting of cortical bone are more resistant to osteoclastic resorption than cancellous blocks. Such resistance is highly desirable especially in esthetic areas with a view to long-term maintenance of a good bone contour. Depending on their thickness and cortical-to-cancellous ratio, blocks can be used either as onlay grafts for full volume augmentation or in the form of thinner veneers or shells. The block graft prevents the overlying soft tissues from collapsing into the defect.

If a bone block graft is not securely fixated, there is a high risk of infection and resorption. Proper fixation of grafts to rule out mechanical mobility and jiggling is essential to bone healing. Block fixation is normally accomplished with titanium screws featuring an external diameter of 1.0–1.5 mm, each of them exerting a holding force of up to 30 kg. Titanium plates, while suitable, are not nor-

mally required for block fixation. Screws for fixation may take the form of either lag screws or positioning screws. Lag screws do not engage the block with their threads, as the gliding hole in the block is slightly wider (Fig 22). The screw presses the block toward the underlying bone as it is tightened, exerting a friction that will stabilize the block. If this type of traction is not wanted, the screw has to engage the block itself, usually by drilling a hole slightly narrower than the external screw diameter into the block (Fig 22). Two screws are used to fixate one bone block, preventing it from rotating. However, a block that has been carefully prepared along with the recipient site can be effectively secured by way of friction even with one single lag screw.

Bone plates are applied to fixate a graft if the underlying bone surface does not offer enough space to anchor lag or positioning screws (Fig 22).

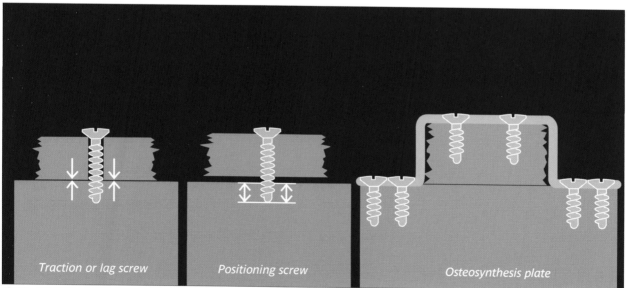

Traction or lag screw   **Positioning screw**   **Osteosynthesis plate**

Fig 22 Lag screws, positioning screw, or plates offer three modes of fixating a block graft. For lag-screw fixation, a large gliding hole is drilled into the bone block, and the screw will engage only the underlying bone but not the block graft. It will press the block against the underlying bone surface and secure it by friction. For positioning-screw fixation, a narrower hole is created, such that the threads will also engage the block graft. Tightening a positioning screw, cannot reduce the distance between the block and the recipient bone surface underneath, will stabilize the former at some distance from the latter.

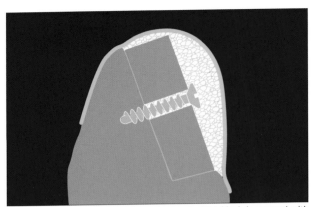

Fig 23a   Onlay technique with a lag screw. The block is covered with
bone substitute material in the periphery.

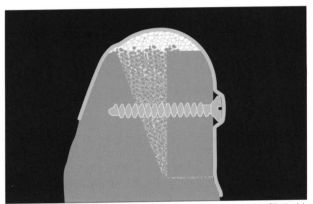

Fig 23b   Shell technique with a positioning screw. The shell is filled with
autologous bone chips. Bone substitutes are used in the periphery.

The lag-screw principle of fixating an onlay block is normally used to expedite integration by establishing intimate contact between the graft and the recipient bone (Fig 23a). Positioning screws can be used to place a block at some distance from the bone surface, acting as a "shell" that establishes a contained space to be filled with autologous particles (Fig 23b).

4.10 Prevention of Premature Graft Resorption

Particulate bone grafts are usually protected with barrier membranes during healing (guided bone regeneration). Experimental studies have demonstrated that a particulate graft will shrink to about half its size unless protected by a membrane during healing (Donos and coworkers 2002). The effect of a membrane on healing has been investigated in several animal studies (Schenk and coworkers 1994; Nyman and Lang 1994). Membrane protection both facilitates the ingrowth of bone cells from the underlying bone tissue and prevents displacement of the graft during healing. Furthermore, a barrier membrane inhibits recruitment of osteoclast precursors, as these cells originate from monocytes in the bloodstream of the overlying soft-tissue flap.

The volume of reconstructed bone remaining after healing depends on a number of factors, including the type of bone or bone substitute used for grafting, the type of membrane applied, the duration of healing, and the strategy that had been adopted to prevent the membrane from collapsing during the healing phase.

While non-resorbable membranes have been shown to produce the most favorable gains in bone volume, they nevertheless involve high rates of complications, one example being membrane exposure due to soft-tissue dehiscence. Exposure of a non-resorbable membrane may create a need for membrane and graft removal tantamount to complete failure of the procedure. Resorbable membranes are less prone to soft-tissue problems leading to their exposure. Any problems of this type, if they do occur, will normally resolve by spontaneous secondary healing with application of local antiseptics. On the downside, these membranes are considered to yield smaller bone gains than their non-resorbable counterparts (Jensen and Terheyden 2009).

Block grafts are commonly used in staged augmentation procedures. Their healing pattern is similar to that of any other free grafts. Although most of the cells do not survive because of the interrupted blood supply, the graft provides an excellent scaffold for ingrowth of cells from adjacent tissues to fully restore vitality and original characteristics of the bone (Urist 1965). Some resorption is needed in this phase to facilitate substitution of non-vital tissue with healed tissue. This mechanism explains why bone grafts tend to shrink during the healing phase (Cordaro and coworkers 2002).

Graft resorption has clinical relevance, since it can interfere with the outcome of the reconstruction. Its rate during healing is influenced by a number of factors, the most important of them being the stability of the graft, origin of the bone used for grafting in terms of endochondral versus intramembranous ossification, the type of bone used for grafting in terms of cortical versus corticocancellous tissue, and soft-tissue healing on top of the graft.

To avoid mobility during healing, block grafts have been secured by the use of lag screws since the late 1980s. As noted earlier, non-rigid fixation will affect healing and result in significant or complete resorption of the block.

Regarding graft origin as a potential modifier of resorption rates, it should be noted that flat bones such as the skull or mandible develop by intramembranous ossification. Their early structures are formed by fibrous connective tissue, which is then replaced by bone. Long bones or the iliac crest, on the other hand, develop by endochondral ossification with cartilage as the primary scaffold for bone deposition.

Also, it has also been demonstrated that bone blocks of a purely cortical nature tend to resorb less than corticocancellous blocks. For the reasons mentioned above, blocks from the mandible or calvaria will normally resorb at a lower rate than iliac-crest grafts.

Soft-tissue dehiscences interfere with the healing of block grafts, promoting resorption and potentially resulting in complete loss of the graft. To avoid such undesirable resorption, it is mandatory to use a surgical technique that will guarantee primary soft-tissue closure over the reconstruction.

Various authors have reported average amounts of bone block resorption varying from 20% to 50% in the absence of complications (Chiapasco and coworkers 2006b). This is not a big clinical problem if the defect can be readily overbuilt or overcontoured. While many clinical situations meet this requirement, others will mandatorily require stable reconstructions. At esthetic sites in particular, even the smallest of volume losses may compromise the outcome.

Another common approach is to combine bone blocks with various bone substitutes and barrier membranes, both of which have been shown to reduce or even elimi-

nate resorption of block grafts (Cordaro and coworkers 2011b; Antoun and coworkers 2001; Wiltfang and coworkers 2012). A prospective randomized trial has substantiated the anti-resorptive effect of barrier membranes (Antoun and coworkers 2001). It is useful to remember that soft-tissue dehiscence and graft exposure may occur more frequently in the presence of a membrane, whether non-resorbable or resorbable.

It should also be noted that graft resorption might be reduced by layering a bone substitute over the bone block (Maiorana and coworkers 2005; von Arx and Buser 2006). Composite grafting with autologous bone blocks, bone substitutes, and barrier membranes is indicated whenever unpredictable resorption of the bone block would jeopardize the outcome (i.e. in the anterior maxilla).

4.11 Simultaneous Versus Staged Augmentation

Bone augmentation may be conducted prior to, or simultaneously with, implant placement. Both approaches are well documented, well accepted, and considered predictable.

The simultaneous approach clearly has its merits. After all, performing all surgery at the same time is less burdensome, costly, and time-consuming. There are also disadvantages, however, including an increased risk of implant exposure if the graft shrinks or is partially resorbed. If much of a bone graft is lost to postoperative wound infection or wound dehiscence, any resultant surface exposure of an osseointegrated implant may turn out untreatable and require a second intervention for implant removal. Simultaneous grafting is more difficult to perform if soft-tissue-level implants are placed in a transmucosal approach, and wound healing is biologically more demanding. The fact that the implant surface will be exposed at least in part to a non-vascularized graft means that delayed osseointegration must be expected in this area. Moreover, exposing a non-vital graft to a non-vital implant surface carries both a risk of infection and a risk of healing by integration in fibrous tissue.

Given these strengths and weaknesses, the simultaneous approach can be recommended in situations meeting the requirements for predictable healing, which needs to be assessed on a case-by-case basis. As a rule, large defects preclude a simultaneous approach. A staged approach is preferred and recommended whenever a bone defect does not allow a good functional and esthetic implant position to be predictably achieved. Other considerations include the form of the bone defect and the location within the dental arch. Self-containing defects can be treated with a simultaneous approach, as the implant is located within the bony envelope in this situation (1/4 defect type—see Table 1 in Chapter 3.4.1). The exposed part of the implant is located further lingually than the adjacent bone walls, allowing the placement and stabilization of a bone graft or substitute. A staged approach should be used with bone defects that require three-dimensional augmentation beyond the existing bony envelope. A staged approach is also required if the bone defect has a vertical component exceeding 1 or 2 millimeters. Other prerequisites for a simultaneous approach include the presence of good local and systemic healing conditions and the absence of severe local and systemic risk factors such as heavy smoking. Furthermore, adequate soft-tissue conditions should be present to ensure predictable coverage of the graft.

4.12 Surgical Planning for Ridge Augmentation in the Esthetic Zone

Clinically, any planning for bone augmentation requires an assessment of the bone volume that is needed to accommodate the position of the prospective implants and prosthetic restoration. A diagnostic wax-up should preferably be created to plan the prosthesis, which can be used for an intraoral try-in and to reach an agreement with the patient about the desired prospective restorative outcome before any treatment steps are undertaken. Alternatively, computer software can be used to perform a virtual wax-up based on imaging data.

The wax-up has a dual function, as it can be transferred to a drilling template. This template should preferably consist of a transparent acrylic resin, and it should indicate both the position and length of the intended prosthetic restoration and the height of the proposed mucosal margin (Fig 24). The implant shoulder of a bone-level implant should be 3 mm below the prospective gingival margin. The bone volume available at the prospective implant sites can be related to the drilling template either indirectly using tomography or directly by ridge mapping under local anesthesia. The most accurate method available at this time is to obtain a cone-beam computed tomography (CBCT) scan with the patient wearing a radiopaque drilling template. Superimposition of the tooth position on the reformatted axial images will reveal the discrepancy between the existing and the required bone volume in all dimensions, yielding needed information about horizontal width and vertical height.

Any bone augmentation in the maxillary anterior segment will normally aim to restore not only function but also esthetics. Creating new bone volume enables the clinician to position an implant in the correct functional and esthetic position. The establishment of a biological width place the soft-tissue margins at constant levels above the bone shoulder. Therefore, bone augmentation can be utilized to adjust and position the marginal mucosa according to the desired prosthodontic plan. This requires predictable and precise bone augmentation techniques and long-term stability of the regenerated bone volume by using appropriate grafting materials.

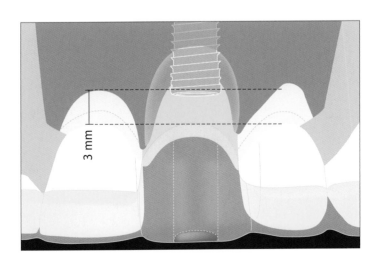

Fig 24 Using a template at the apical crown margin, the required amount of reconstruction can be directly measured.

4.13 Augmentation Protocols

4.13.1 Dehiscence Defects and Fenestrations

As the focus of this volume is mainly on the staged approach of reconstructing the alveolar bone prior to implant placement, we shall only briefly address the simultaneous approach of treating small bone defects at the time of implant placement. Dehiscence and fenestration defects may occur whenever an existing bone volume is too small to completely surround an implant upon insertion (Figs 25 and 26e-f). Dehiscence refers to a bone defect at the crest of the alveolar ridge. Defects of this type may occur at the shoulder of an implant due to the rounded form of the alveolar crest, and usually they are encountered on the facial side (1/4 defect type—see Table 1 and Fig 38). The roughened portion of the implant surface may thus become exposed and colonized by bacteria from the peri-implant sulcus via a long junctional epithelium unless a grafting procedure is performed to augment the bone. Fenestration defects, by contrast, occur at implant sites with undercuts or concavities of the alveolar ridge. While the implant shoulder remains fully covered by bone in this situation, exposure is seen at some point of the implant body at a more apical level (Fig 25).

Simultaneous bone augmentation of dehiscence defects should only be considered if they present as a self-containing type of defect. Otherwise, a staged approach is recommended.

A well-designed full-thickness flap should be elevated that offers good access to the defect and a good view. The preferred incision line is of the midcrestal linear type extending to the neighboring teeth as a sulcular incision. A vertical incision should be used to release tension.

The cortical plate around the implant dehiscence is cleared of soft-tissue remnants and perforated with a small round bur. The cambium layer on the outer bone surface is also removed. A bone trap can be used to collect the bone chips produced, as well as the chips from the previous preparation of the implant bed. More material can be collected from the cortical bone surrounding the defect with a bone scraper. Thin and unstable layers of cortical bone over the implant, rather than leaving

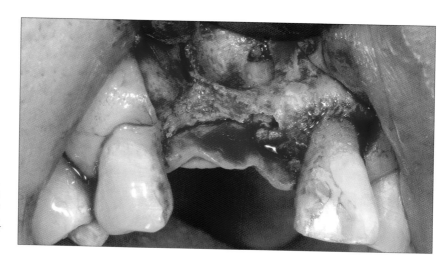

Fig 25   An implant osteotomy has been prepared. While the marginal bone is intact, a visible fenestration has occurred more apically due to the steep concavity of the buccal bone. Guided bone regeneration is the treatment of choice.

them in situ where they might pose a risk of necrosis and infection, are removed and mixed with the particulate graft. Then, as a first layer for grafting, the autologous bone chips are distributed over the implant surface up to the implant shoulder, followed by a second layer of bone substitute at least 2 mm thick.

This second layer is finally covered with a resorbable collagen membrane, which does not usually require fixation. The goal in selecting and cutting the membrane should be to cover all defect areas and the graft completely. The membrane may be extended below the palatal or the lingual flap. It will adhere to the site once blood from the underlying grafted area soaks through. While the membrane may also cover the alveolar bone of the neighboring teeth, it should not protrude through the sulcus on repositioning the flap. A double-layer technique is usually employed to place the membrane, both to stabilize the reconstruction and to decelerate membrane resorption for an optimized barrier function (Buser 2009).

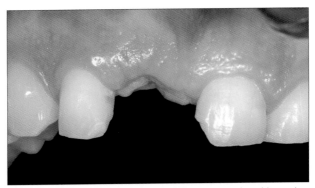

Fig 26a   Young man with a thick gingival biotype presenting with an edentulous space (trauma-induced loss of a central upper incisor) and coronal fracture of the adjacent tooth.

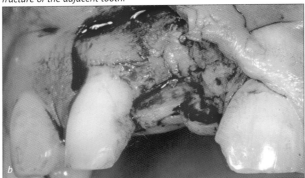 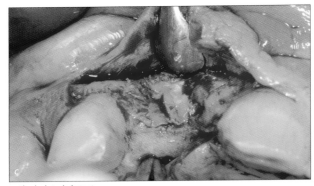

Figs 26b-c   Flap elevation reveals a moderate defect of the buccal plate. The cortical plate is intact.

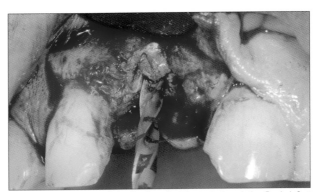

Fig 26d   Preparation of the implant bed is started and the final defect anticipated.

The flap is then released to achieve passive repositioning, using interrupted sutures and horizontal mattress sutures to close the site. Recent publications suggest that transmucosal healing may also be a viable option in the esthetic zone if simultaneous bone augmentation is performed. Submerged healing, while involving a second surgical stage, may facilitate soft-tissue management (Hämmerle and Lang 2001; Cordaro and coworkers 2012b).

A typical clinical case in which this approach was used is shown in Figure 26a-m.

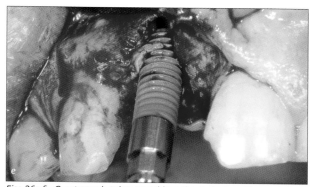 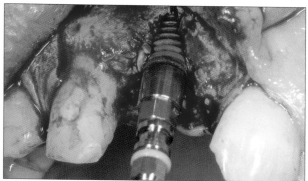

Figs 26e-f   Great care is taken to achieve the desired position and depth of implant insertion, using a bone-level implant in this specific case. Once inserted, a horizontal defect mimicking a vertical defect is apparent. More than half of the buccal implant surface is not covered by bone.

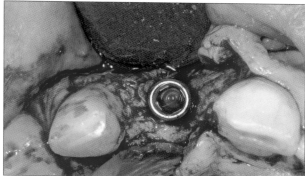

Fig 26g   This occlusal view clearly reveals the self-containing nature of the defect, since the alveolar bone of the adjacent teeth is located several millimeters further buccally than the defect and will support the bone substitute.

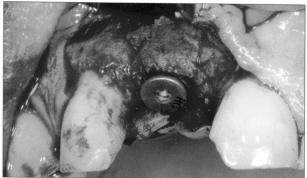 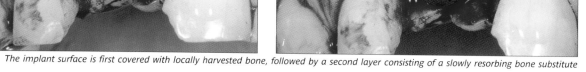

Figs 26h-i   The implant surface is first covered with locally harvested bone, followed by a second layer consisting of a slowly resorbing bone substitute (DBBM).

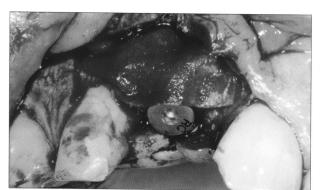

Fig 26j   The entire reconstruction is covered with a double layer of collagen membrane.

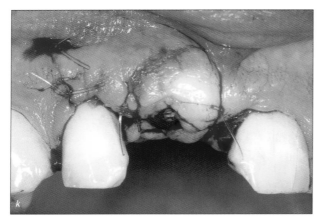

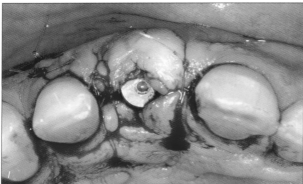

Figs 26k-l A semi-submerged healing protocol is used. This occlusal view clearly displays the overcorrection of the horizontal defect.

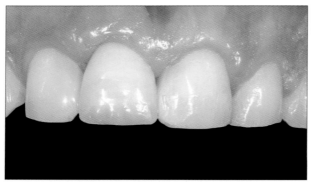

Fig 26m Postoperative view. This augmentation technique may be adequate—if conditions are favorable—to achieve a predictable outcome even in the esthetic zone

4.13.2 Onlay Graft for Lateral Ridge Augmentation (Staged Procedure)

A ridge too narrow to accommodate dental implants can essentially be addressed by two distinctive strategies of staged surgery, one consisting of ridge expansion, the other of onlay grafting using block grafts, membrane-protected grafts, or guided bone regeneration (GBR).

The procedure of horizontal augmentation with an onlay block graft is started by performing a midcrestal incision and extending it to the adjacent teeth/implants as a sulcular incision. A flap is elevated and the recipient bone exposed to assess the required block size. A sterile piece of paper (e.g. of a suture package) may be used to create a block-size template, and the selected approach to harvesting the block should allow for chip collection in a bone trap.

Next, the surface of the recipient bone is cleared of soft-tissue remnants, preferably by using a large round bur. A very small round bur can be used to perforate the cortical surface of the recipient bone to gain access to the marrow cavity. These chips may be collected as well.

The block graft is then fitted into the recipient defect, usually preceded by removing bone from the recipient site to open its marrow cavity. Once the block has been fixated, it is contoured with a round bur while, again collecting the chips. The block should stand as a space-preserving structure in the center of the augmentation, preferably forming the buccal bone plate for the prospective implants. The dimension and position of the block required to achieve this can be controlled by a surgical guide, which should be prepared before the augmentation surgery.

A mimimum of 2 mm bone thickness facial to the prospective dental implant should be achieved by the augmentation.

A block harvested from the mandibular ramus will usually be 3 to 5 mm thick, such that a ridge of 4 mm can be expanded to a width of 7 to 9 mm. Ridges thinner than that (down to 1 mm in width, as exemplified by the typical appearance of knife-edge ridges in posterior mandibles or atrophic edentulous ridges in anterior maxillae) are managed with the shell technique, which is discussed later and can also be used to compensate for vertical deficits.

Block grafts may be covered with barrier membranes and bone chips or a slowly resorbing bone substitute. This will reduce resorption.

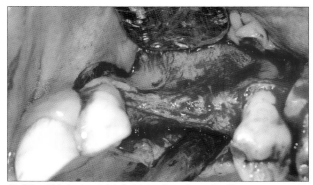

Fig 27a   This horizontal defect is too large for a simultaneous augmentation procedure. The canine and the first premolar are missing.

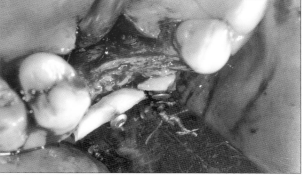

Fig 27b   A block harvested from the ramus is divided in two and adapted to the recipient site. Two screws are used to stabilize the grafts.

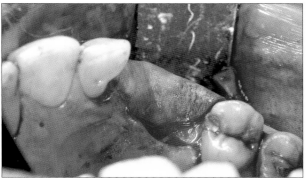

Fig 27c   Bone chips and a collagen membrane are used to cover the graft. The membrane is tucked under the palatal flap.

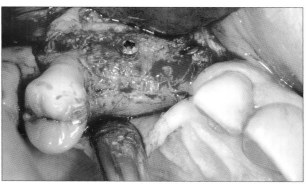

Fig 27d   Re-entry after 4 months. Note the good outcome of bone augmentation.

For membrane protection, a resorbable collagen membrane is placed over the block and tucked under the lingual or palatal flap. A mixed bone graft is prepared from the remaining autologous chips, DBBM, and autologous blood. This particulate material is then used to cover the entire block and create a smooth shape that will minimize the irregularities of the reconstructed bone profile.

A prerequisite for safe healing is to achieve a soft-tissue closure that involves no tension and is impermeable to fluids. It is recommended to use fine sutures that will exhibit a low tendency for plaque accumulation (e.g. 5-0 atraumatic monofilament) using atraumatic needles. Long incisions are usually closed with a few mattress sutures that relieve the tension and unfold the wound edges, followed by single interrupted sutures placed in between. Overly short intervals between the sutures should be avoided because healing of the wound edges will only take place between them but not underneath. Even finer sutures (e.g. 6-0) should be selected for releasing incisions in the esthetic zone.

Figure 27a-e illustrates a block-graft procedure for horizontal augmentation in a partially edentulous patient.

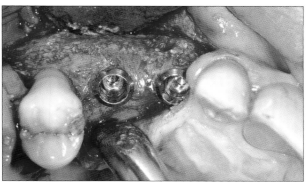

Fig 27e   Two implants have been placed into the reconstructed ridge. Note the adequate width of the bone walls on the facial and palatal surfaces of the implants.

4.13.3 Ridge Splitting for Lateral Ridge Augmentation

An alternative method of augmenting a narrow ridge is by ridge splitting instead of onlay grafting. This technique can be applied in selected cases. It requires that the alveolar ridge has two cortical plates separated by a layer of cancellous bone in a preoperative CBCT image. This is a situation that is normally confined to alveolar ridges featuring an orofacial thickness of more than 4 mm. Narrower ridges are usually associated with a thin or nonexistent cancellous compartment. If that is the case, onlay grafting is the augmentation method of choice (Figs 28a-d).

Ridge splitting carries a risk of unpredictable vertical resorption of the outer bone lamella by reducing or obliterating blood supply to that structure. Ridge splitting can be performed simultaneously with implant placement. The only way to obtain primary stability in this scenario is by engaging the bone at apical region of the implant. This may result in reduced primary stability of the implant, as the buccal bone plate is no longer rigid. In selected cases, it may be possible to stabilize the mobilized buccal plate with bone screws if required.

It is advisable to perform the splitting with minimal flap reflection to expose only the crestal region of the ridge. Partial flap reflection may reduce resorption by preserving vascularization of the split buccal bone lamella. Better vascularization of cortical bone is present in the maxilla due to multiple periosteal branches in the cortical bone. Clinically, the ridge is opened through a midline crestal incision. A full-thickness flap of only a few millimeters is detached on the buccal and lingual sides. If required, the flap can be apically extended as a split-thickness flap, leaving the periosteal blood flow intact.

This will expose the coronal aspect of the ridge to view, and its buccolingual width can be measured.

Once the flap is raised, a linear groove is prepared in the middle of the ridge with rotating burs or a piezosurgery device. Subsequently an osteotome chisel with a tiny blade is used to deepen this linear slit. Careful tapping with a mallet will gently advance the chisel into the cancellous compartment, using the lingual or palatal cortical bone for guidance. To achieve harmonious widening of the ridge, this osteotomy should be created slightly deeper than the planned implant length. In hard and brittle bone, vertical releasing bone cuts can be added by carefully palpation beneath the soft tissue with the chisel. Care should be taken not to perforate the mucosa during this maneuver. In the more elastic maxillary bone, these vertical cuts can usually be avoided. Piezosurgery devices are helpful in preserving the mucosa due to their property of selectively cutting bone rather than soft tissue.

After completion of the bone cuts, the bone slit is slowly widened. Metal wedges are driven into the slit, which are available from dental instrument manufacturers. Other options include the use of condensation instruments or a root elevator. The aim is to gently bend the outer lamella in a buccal direction while leaving the palatal (or lingual) cortical plate intact and stable. In the maxilla, this can be accomplished without causing a fracture if handled patiently. In the mandible, the bone may be so hard and brittle as to break. The maneuver is repeated until the crestal ridge has been sufficiently widened to accommodate the implants. These should be placed slightly deeper (below the crest) than usual to compensate for the resorption and mild height reduction of the buccal bone that may follow. If the ridge splitting is conducted in a staged approach, bone substitute particles

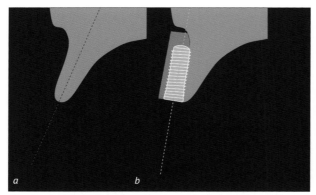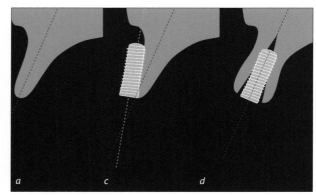

Figs 28a-d   This scenario of a knife-edge ridge illustrates the prosthetic outcomes attainable by either block grafting or bone splitting. Ridge splitting has the limitation of requiring an implant position inside the axis of the split (within the cancellous compartment), which may not coincide with the prosthetic axis. The implant axis could be adjusted more freely with an onlay graft. (a) Initial situation. (b) Block graft. (c) Divergence between the ideal axis offered by block grafting and the less-than-ideal axis resulting from ridge splitting.(d) Splitting technique and prosthetic axis of the inserted implant.

rather than the implant can be packed into the gap to preserve the buccolingual width that has been gained.

Soft-tissue closure is performed next. Because the crest is now wider than before, complete adaptation of the flaps cannot be achieved unless the flap has been completely mobilized beforehand. Since this is not recommended, the soft tissues are adapted with interrupted sutures but not firmly closed. Open gaps can be closed with small pieces of collagen fleece.

A somewhat higher level of surgical skill and experience is needed for flapless ridge splitting compared to conventional bone grafting. An epiperiosteal flap would be one alternative but is difficult to prepare at marginal levels and would destroy the natural vascular network of the flap. Another alternative would be to use a full-thickness flap, which has the advantage of offering good vision but detaches the split lamella from its soft-tissue pedicle. It is also possible to use mixed flaps, like combining a full-thickness design at the coronal level with a split-thickness design at the apical level.

The main indication for ridge splitting is to expand a horizontally reduced ridge in the maxilla and take advantage of the elastic and cancellous quality of this bone and its peripheral type of blood perfusion. Splitting a narrow mandibular ridge is possible but technically more difficult due to the brittle, thicker, and more cortical nature of this bone. Blood perfusion in the mandible occurs centrally, with less blood flowing through the thin periosteal branches than in the maxilla. A flapless approach in the maxilla offers the benefit that even small bone fragments remain attached to the periosteum and are contained by the intact soft-tissue envelope. On balance, ridge expansion via bone splitting is effective but does have its limitations both in terms of anatomic requirements and with regard to a clinician's surgical skills. Onlay block grafting, with addition of particulated grafts and a membrane for protection, is the more versatile and widely used approach. The procedure it involves is better documented in the literature and less technique sensitive than ridge splitting (Aghaloo and Moy 2007). Also, block grafts are more predictable in terms of involving less inadvertent resorption than buccally split lamellae following ridge expansion (see also Chapter 6.12).

Figure 29 illustrates two ridge-splitting procedures in the maxilla (Figs 29a-g) and in the mandible (Figs 30a-l).

Acknowledgments (Figs 29a-g)

Prosthodontic procedures
Dr. Kai Schaumburg – Kassel, Germany

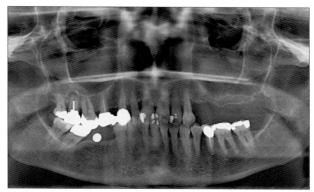

Fig 29a Panoramic radiograph of an initial situation characterized by a free-end situation in the left maxilla without a vertical bone deficit (2/4 defect).

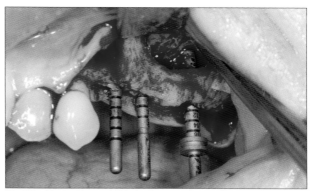

Fig 29b Vertical bone deficit in the posterior maxilla combined with a horizontal deficit in the first premolar region. A preparation of the sinus membrane has already been performed. The pilot holes have been drilled according to the drilling template.

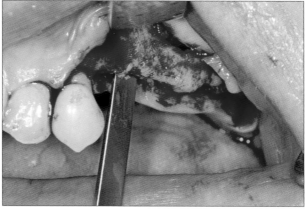

Fig 29c A longitudinal slit has been cut into the crestal part of the ridge with a small Lindemann bur. A flat osteotome (chisel) is inserted and gently pushed forward with a mallet. The osteotomy is prepared slightly deeper than the prospective implant level.

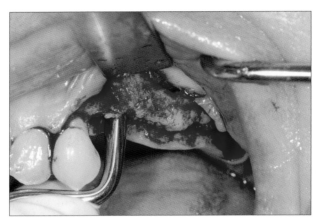

Fig 29d   A root elevator is used to gently mobilize the buccal bone plate outward. This should be done very slowly and carefully to stay within the elastic limit of the bone and not risk complete fracture and detachment of the buccal bone plate.

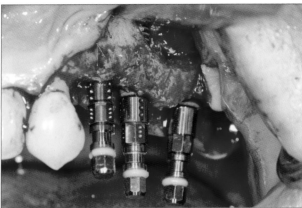

Fig 29e   Bone-level implants 4.1 mm in diameter (Straumann AG, Basel, Switzerland) are inserted in the premolar region. A 4.8-mm implant (Straumann) is used at the molar site. Primary stability is limited due to the reduced stability of the buccal bone

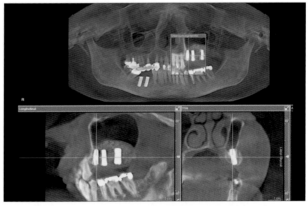

Fig 29f   Postoperative CBCT scan demonstrating an adequate ridge width (with bone buccal to the implant at site 24) and an effective outcome of sinus floor augmentation

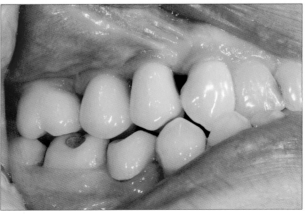

Fig 29g   Final prosthesis.

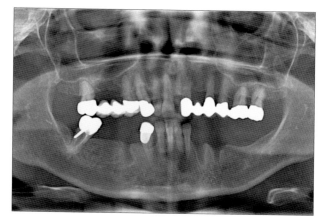

Fig 30a   Panoramic radiograph of an initial situation prior to implant surgery. Teeth 33, 34, and 44 had been extracted 6 months previously. The current procedure included extraction of teeth 43 and 47 with immediate placement of implants.

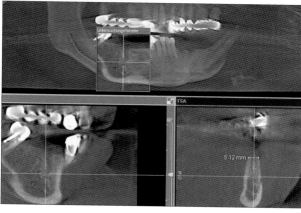

Fig 30b   An average ridge width of approximately 5 mm was noted prior to ridge splitting.

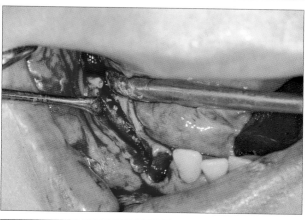

Fig 30c   A flap was carefully elevated from the top of the ridge via an accurate median incision into the linea alba. In an effort not to interfere with the vascular supply to the mandible, the flap was reflected only slightly. The bony ridge was split with a small Lindemann bur. Vertical osteotomies were created before site 44 and behind site 46.

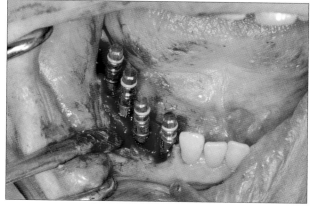

Fig 30d   A chisel was used to separate both cortical plates and the splitting buccal lamella was bent outward, taking care not to detach or fracture the lingual bone plate, followed by simultaneous placement of implants. These were inserted slightly below the level of the buccal cortical plate to compensate for vertical resorption of the splitting lamella. The implant at site 43 was placed into a fresh extraction socket.

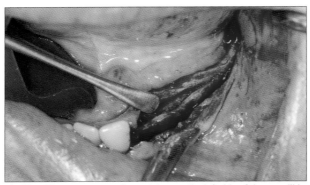

Fig 30e   The same approach was taken on the left side of the mandible. Here the splitting lamella had already been bent outward without detaching or fracturing the lingual bone plate.

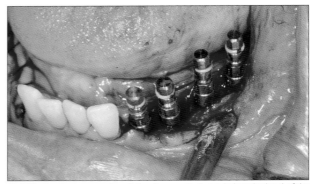

Fig 30f   Implants were placed simultaneously 1 mm below the level of the splitting buccal lamella.

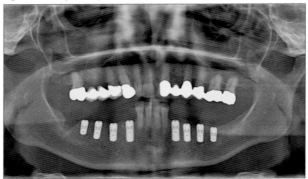

Fig 30g   Panoramic radiograph obtained after implant placement.

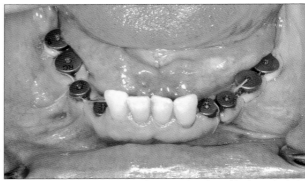

Fig 30h   Surgical implant uncovering. Note that the residual attached gingiva is split and distributed evenly around the implants.

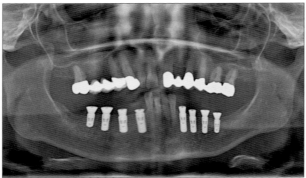

Fig 30i   Panoramic radiograph obtained after implant uncovering.

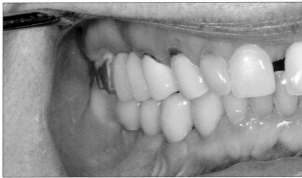

Fig 30j   Follow-up 1 year after delivery (right side). The tissues are stable

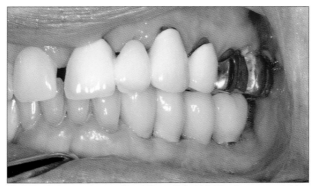

Fig 30k   Follow-up 1 year after delivery (left side). The tissues are stable.

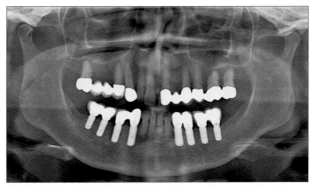

Fig 30l   Panoramic radiograph obtained 1 year after prosthetic delivery.

4.13.4 Vertical Ridge Augmentation

Vertical augmentation is indicated if a ridge has insufficient vertical height to accommodate implants of the required length. Procedures of this type are typically performed in free-end situations in atrophic posterior mandibles with a bone height of less than 10 mm above the nerve. Situations with more than 10 mm of bone height can usually be managed with implants 8 mm in length. Shorter implants may be considered but may involve reduced success rates (Telleman and coworkers 2011).

As a rule, procedures for vertical augmentation are more challenging than those for horizontal augmentation and are normally performed in a staged approach (Rocchietta and coworkers 2008). Reasons for the increased risk they pose include a higher level of soft-tissue tension resulting from wound closure and mechanical loading of the grafts by oral function.

Onlay block grafting is the traditional method of vertical augmentation, and one that offers predictable outcomes (Proussaefs and Lozada 2005). Eligible materials for such grafting include an iliac corticocancellous block, a cranial cortical graft, or mandibular bone. Bone of ample height and width to deal with cases of extensive edentulism can be harvested from the iliac wing. The graft can be planned and contoured to restore the ideal height and width. For a large onlay graft, the buccal and lingual soft tissues need to be detached and mobilized, which commonly results in relocation of the attached mucosa. Free gingival grafts and vestibuloplasties are often required as secondary procedures to reconstruct the keratinized mucosa around the implant.

A significant problem of vertical onlay blocks is vertical bone resorption, which is related in part to the extensive soft-tissue mobilization that these procedures require.

At times, the resorption may be rather unpredictable and continue over years. If the definitive implants were placed simultaneously with the grafting procedure, such persistent resorption may lead to esthetic and functional failure as implant bodies become exposed to the oral cavity. For this reason, the recommended (and almost exclusively used) way of performing vertical augmentation is to take a staged approach.

Vertical onlay procedures can also be conducted similarly to the one described for staged horizontal augmentation, with guided bone regeneration (GBR) using an onlay bone block. Alternative options include the use of a reinforced polytetrafluoroethylene (PTFE) membrane in conjunction with supporting tenting screws or even a simultaneous approach that utilizes the implants themselves as tenting poles to augment height deficiencies of up to 7 mm (Simion and coworkers 2007).

4.13.5 Shell Technique for Vertical Augmentation

Atrophic ridges presenting with a reduced height combined with a knife-edge morphology can be treated by fixating an autologous cortical block in an overlapping fashion to create a "shell" on their buccal aspect (Figs 31a-m). Fixation is accomplished not with lag screws but with positioning screws. The upper edge of the block should be positioned to serve as the buccal bone plate of the prospective implants. The idea is to create an open space between the ridge and the shell-like bone graft, which should be filled with autologous bone. The external layers can be covered with a mixed graft and a resorbable collagen membrane. Care should be taken not to overcorrect the deficiency vertically while at the same time maintaining at least 7 mm of interocclusal clearance for the prosthodontic work.

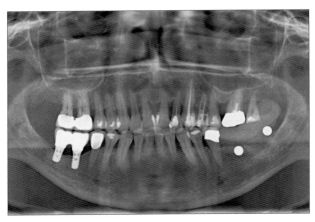

Fig 31a   Panoramic radiograph. Freeend situation on the left side of the mandible, characterized by a horizontal—and slightly vertical—bone deficiency (3/4 defect).

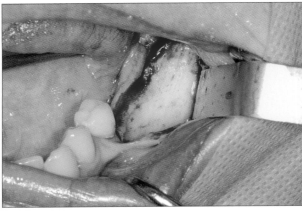

Fig 31b   Teeth 36 and 37 are missing. A fullthickness flap is reflected, using a midcrestal incision with a small retromolar releasing incision 45° toward the ascending ramus and a sulcular incision at tooth 35. The lingual soft tissues are detached, including the retromolar area. Usually, the lingual periosteum is sufficiently elastic to be mobilized passively.

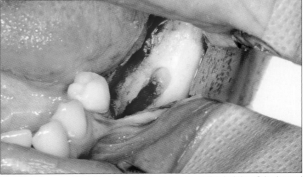

Fig 31c   A groove is drilled 1 cm below the prospective height of the buccal bone shoulder.

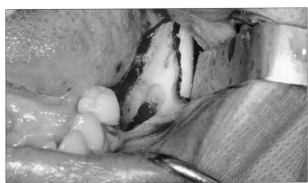

Fig 31d   A bone block 2×1 cm in size is harvested form the external oblique ridge. Bone chips are collected with a bone trap.

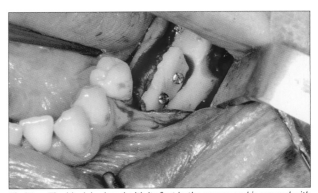

Fig 31e   The block is placed with its foot in the groove and is secured with two positioning screws.

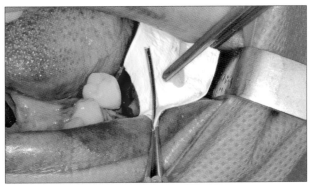

Fig 31f   A resorbable collagen membrane is cut and a tongue of the membrane placed under the lingual flap.

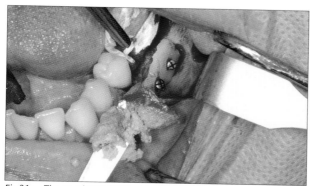

Fig 31g   The membrane is secured underneath the lingual flap. The space behind the block is filled with autologous bone chips.

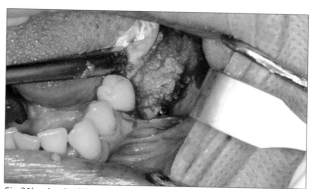

Fig 31h   A mixed bone graft (DBBM and bone chips in equal parts) is placed in 2 mm vertical and horizontal excess lingually and over the graft.

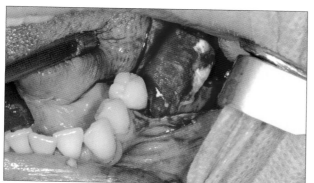

Fig 31i   The membrane is folded over the graft and the flap mobilized to safely cover the graft.

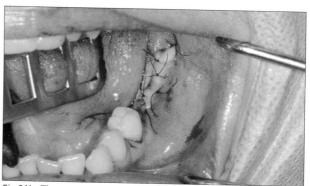

Fig 31j   The wound is closed with two mattress sutures (4-0) and interrupted sutures (5-0).

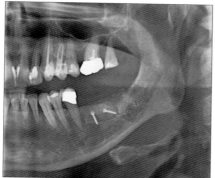

Fig 31k   Postoperative panoramic radiograph.

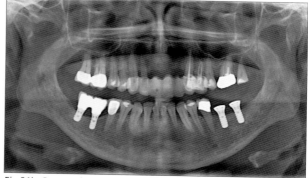

Fig 31l   Panoramic radiograph following implant installation 4 months after augmentation.

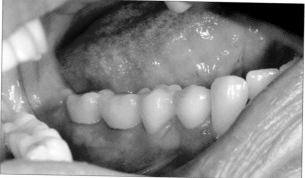

Fig 31m   Final prosthesis.

4.13.6 Interpositional Graft for Vertical Augmentation

A relatively new development to overcome the problems of vertical onlay grafts in 4/4 defects (i.e. extensive mobilization of soft tissues and unpredictable bone resorption) is by an interpositional graft, also known as a "sandwich graft" (Figs 32b-c). This approach leaves the soft tissues on the oral side of the midcrestal incision attached to the crestal bone segment. No lateral shift of the mucogingival junction occurs.

This technique should only be performed by experienced surgeons due to its high complexity and the possibility of severe complications.

A midcrestal incision is performed and a full-thickness flap reflected. In the mandible, the mental foramen is exposed and the nerve protected, while the lingual soft tissues remain attached to the bone. One horizontal bone cut and two vertical ones are performed to prepare a box-style bone segment. After the osteotomy, the crestal bone segment remains attached to the lingual soft-tissue pedicle. In the posterior mandible, the horizontal bone split needs to end well above the alveolar nerve. At least 4 to 5 mm of residual bone height are required above the nerve. If these conditions are not met, the procedure should be abandoned in favor of an onlay graft from the iliac crest. Osteotomies of this type performed in the interforaminal area of the mandible are possible below the level of the mandibular nerves. In the posterior mandible, the lingual periosteum is usually very thin and does not limit the height of elevation of the seg-ment. In the anterior maxilla, the attainable gain in bone height is limited by the rigidity of the palatal soft tissue and cannot exceed 2 to 4 mm. An alternative to interpositional grafting in this situation would be distraction osteogenesis.

Osteosynthesis plates are used to immobilize the pedicled bone segment at its required vertical position to allow placing implants of ideal restorative length and position in a secondstage procedure. A box-style gap opens between the segments, which borders on an open bone-marrow cavity on two sides. This space offers excellent conditions for vascularization of the graft and bone healing. It can be filled with a mixture of bone substitute and bone chips that were collected with a bone trap from the osteotomy site. On the buccal side, a periosteal incision with mobilization of the flap is required. A collagen membrane may be applied over the buccal interpositional gap.

4.13.7 Swinging Interpositional Graft for Vertical and Horizontal Augmentation

This variation of the sandwich technique is used on 3/4 ridge defects (Figs 32b and 33a-i). It works on the principle that the oblique outer plate of a narrow ridge can be swung upward until it stands horizontally. A similar contained defect type opens below, which can be filled with a mixed bone graft. The segment remains attached to the lingual soft tissues and is stabilized with titanium plates for 4 months.

Figs 31a-e   Three alternatives (a-c) to onlay grafting (d-e) for vertical augmentation.

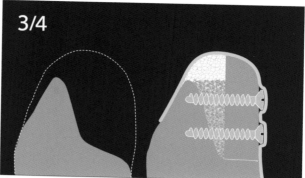

Fig 32a   Shell technique.

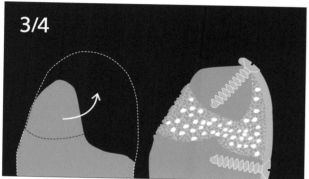

Fig 32b   Swinging interpositional graft.

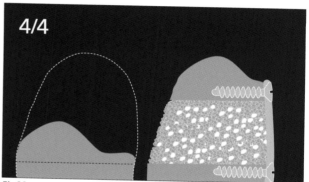

Fig 32c   Staged interpositional graft (alternative: distraction osteogenesis).

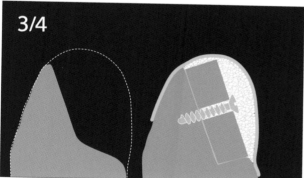

Fig 32d   Onlay technique 3/4 ridge defect.

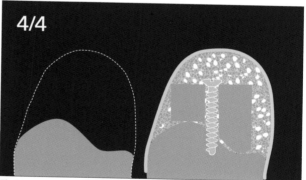

Fig 32e   Onlay technique 4/4 ridge defect.

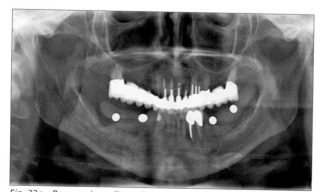

Fig 33a   Panoramic radiograph. A combined horizontal and vertical deficit (3/4 defect)

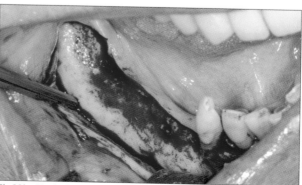

Fig 33b   Vertical defect. A midcrestal incision is used with the lingual soft tissues remaining attached.

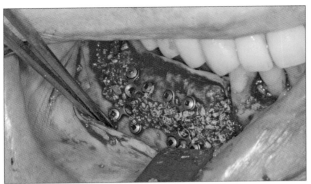

Fig 33c   After completion of the osteotomy, the segment is swung upward and secured in its correct prosthetic position relative to the opposing dentition. The interpositional space is filled with grafting material mixed from DBBM and autologous bone chips in equal parts.

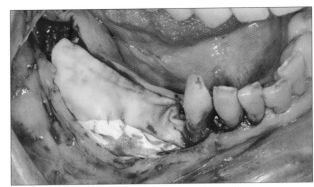

Fig 33d   The defect is covered with a resorbable membrane.

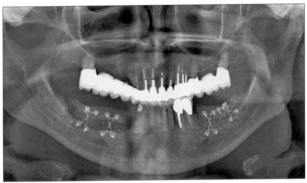

Fig 33e   Postoperative panoramic radiograph.

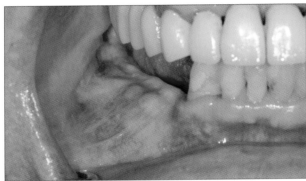

Fig 33f   Situation after 4 months. The graft has healed. Its prosthetic position relative to the opposing dentition is favorable.

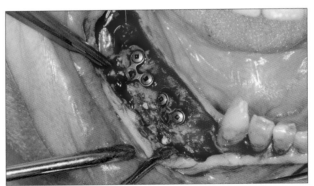

Fig 33g   The segment is stable. The plates have been removed.

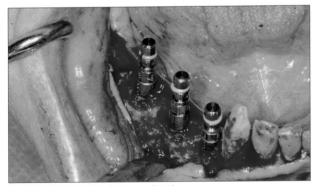

Fig 33h   Bone-level implants are placed.

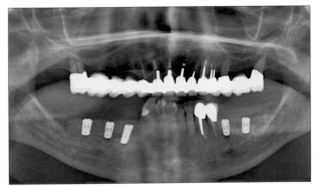

Fig 33i   Panoramic radiograph after implant installation.

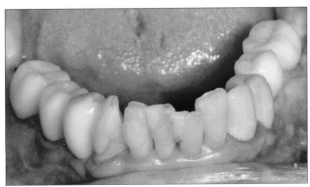

Fig 33j   Final prosthesis.

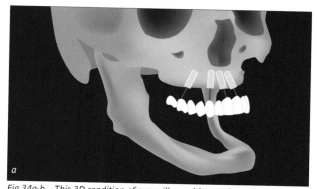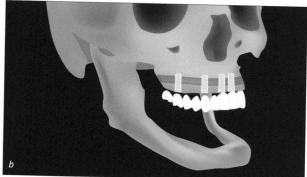

Fig 34a-b   This 3D rendition of a maxilla—with superimposition of a radiographic template—illustrates the angulated position and crossbites associated with ridge atrophy in the maxilla.

4.13.8 Interpositional Graft for Vertical Augmentation in the Maxilla (Le Fort I Level)

Le Fort I interpositional grafting takes advantage of the possibility to simultaneously adjust the sagittal and vertical occlusal position of the alveolar crest with simultaneous grafting performed at the same time.

The Le Fort I osteotomy was originally designed for orthognathic procedures and has been successfully applied to edentulous atrophic jaws (Bell and coworkers 1977). A Le Fort I interpositional graft can be used to move the anterior ridge and expand it into its ideal sagittal and vertical restorative position. In this way, implant-supported fixed restorations can be implemented in cases of bone atrophy. The technique is indicated in cases of mild atrophy like the ones seen after periodontal bone loss (Cawood class IV) but also in severe (class V) and extreme (class VI) cases (Cawood and Howell 1988).

Maxillary ridge atrophy will normally proceed centripetally. Both the height of the crest and its anterior projection are reduced in the process, resulting in a pseudo-class-III relationship associated with lack of support for the lip and nose. Any implants placed in this situation usually have to be tilted by approximately 30 degrees to make them project over the opposing dentition. To make things worse, the superstructure would have to consist of long crowns or a removable denture with artificial replacement of lost tissues (Figs 34a-b and 35). Le Fort I interpositional grafting reverses such displacement of the maxillary crest, such that bone can be created for normally positioned (non-tilted) implants and fixed prostheses with optimal crown lengths. Also, the procedure will reestablish adequate support for the soft tissues of the lip and nose. The edentulous maxilla receives its blood supply from the palate and the posterior soft-tissue pedicle of the throat. This vascularization is not jeopardized by detaching the vestibular

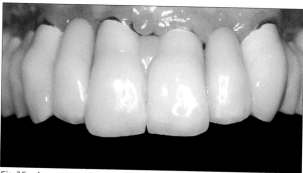

Fig 35   A way to address situations of non-favourable vertical bone loss is to add a pink ceramic flange (epithesis) to the prosthesis or to fabricate long crowns (as shown here). This involves placement of the implants in compromised positions (e.g. protruded by 30°).

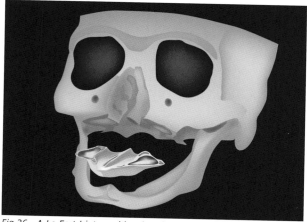

Fig 36   A Le Fort I interpositional graft according to Bell and coworkers (1977) as shown in this drawing can be used to augment maxillae that are extremely atrophic (Cawood classes V and VI). The method is also used for vertical augmentation to eliminate the need for a removable denture in moderately atrophic cases (Cawood class IV).

soft tissues and subsequent downfracture. Furthermore, the mucosa of the nasal floor and the sinus floors can be kept intact in the downfractured maxilla. The resultant defect is closed and contained and can subsequently be treated with particulated grafts and/or bone substitutes, grafting and expanding the resorbed crest from the inside. Titanium plates are used for stabilization once the correct prosthetic position of the maxilla has been established (Fig 36).

Access to the maxilla is created through a midcrestal incision into the linea alba from the second-molar site to the contralateral side. The osteotomy is started by preparing sinus windows bilaterally to elevate the sinus mucosa (Figs. 37a-b).

The next step is to prepare the mucosa of the nasal floor carefully on both sides, followed by a horizontal osteotomy involving the canine buttress and the posterior lateral sinus wall. A chisel is used to cut the medial sinus wall, a septum chisel to detach the nasal septum from the nasal floor, and a curved chisel to separate the pterygoid process from the maxilla. Then the maxilla is downfractured and gently mobilized.

The degree to which the anterior ridge can be advanced and lengthened with this approach will depend on the restoration-driven surgical plan. Titanium bone plates are used for ridge fixation in the canine and the zygomatic buttresses. It is advisable to reinforce the canine buttress with iliac blocks grafts, bridging the osteotomy gap to ensure that occlusal stability will be reestablished after 4 months. Also, small strips of iliac bone may be used to reinforce the crest if required. Finally the interpositional gap—including the sinus and nasal floors—is filled with a mixed graft of DBBM and autologous bone particles (Figs 38a-g; see also chapter 6.12, Figs 1 to 17).

A less extensive type of Le Fort I osteotomy would be to create a partial segmental interpositional osteotomy in the anterior maxilla, for example to address periodontal bone loss associated with the anterior dentition. The vertical movement attainable with this specific procedure is limited by the rigidity of the palatal soft tissues to merely a few millimeters.

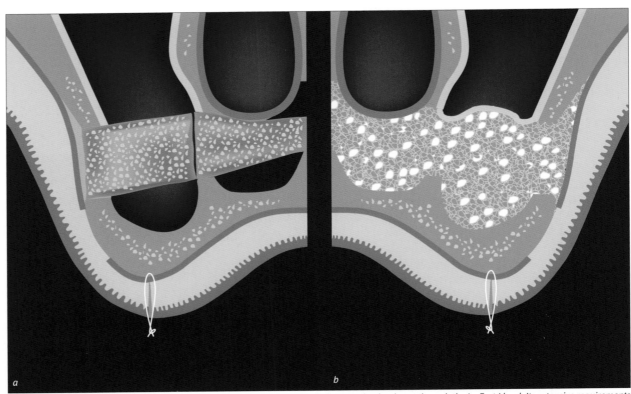

a *b*

Figs 37a-b Old (left) and new (right) techniques. The originally described technique used a simple cut through the Le Fort I level. Its extensive requirements for bone-block grafting were considerably burdensome for patients. The contemporary technique uses bilateral elevation of the sinus and nasal floors, resulting in a closed and contained defect that can be filled with bone substitutes to reduce the need for iliac-bone harvesting.

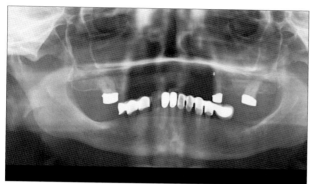

Fig 38a   Panoramic radiograph. Marked bone deficit in the anterior maxilla, due in part to a combination syndrome resulting from the hard opposing dentition.

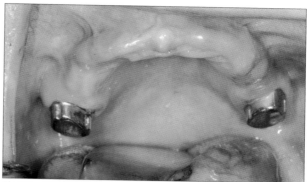

Fig 38b   Clinical view of an edentulous maxilla, characterized by moderate atrophy with a significant anterior deficit and a flappy ridge (Cawood class IV).

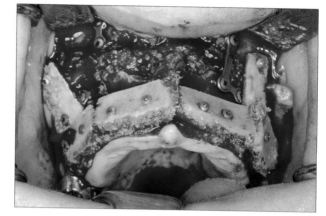

Fig 38c   A midcrestal incision is performed—along with two vertical releasing incisions 45° behind the tuberosity—to expose the facial bone wall of the maxilla including the maxillary nerves at the piriform opening. Following bilateral elevation of the sinus and nasal floors, the interpositional gap is filled with a mixed bone graft (DBBM and bone chips in equal parts). Plates are used to fixate the maxilla at the canine site, carefully adjusting the height of the crest and its sagittal interocclusal relationship. An iliac-bone block is applied to restore the canine buttress and bridge the interpositional gap. Additional strips of iliac bone are used to reinforce the ridge horizontally.

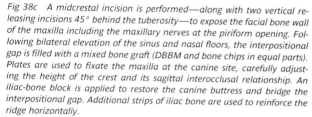

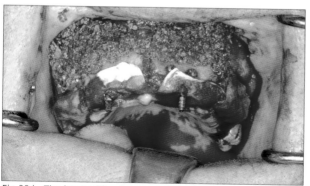

Fig 38d   The interpositional space and the buccal space between the framework of the iliac bone strips is filled with mixed bone graft. Provisional implants are placed into the pristine bone.

Fig 38e   Postoperative panoramic radiograph.

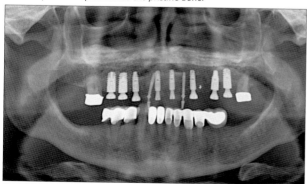

Fig 38f   Panoramic radiograph after surgical re-entry for implant exposure.

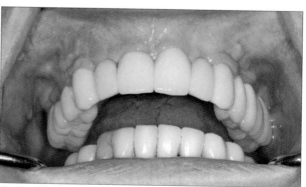

Fig 38g   Fixed restoration in place.

4.14 Guidelines for Selecting the Appropriate Augmentation Protocol

The formulation of a treatment plan in medicine and dentistry should be guided by a logical process. Decisions for treatment should always be based on precise diagnostics, an appraisal of outcomes to be expected with different treatment options that may be available, and an evaluation of whether the ultimately chosen strategy is appropriate for use in a specific patient or whether local or systemic factors in that individual may suggest otherwise.

As described previously in Chap 2.2, the systematic review of Milincovic and Cordaro (2013) reported that only a few studies of augmentation techniques characterized the baseline defect. Therefore, well-defined evidence-based protocols for clinicians to select the most appropriate technique for each specific clinical situation are still unavailable. We endeavor to provide such definitions based on three sources of knowledge:

- Classification of defects (Fig 39).
- Evidence from the literature, however limited.
- The present authors' expert opinions.

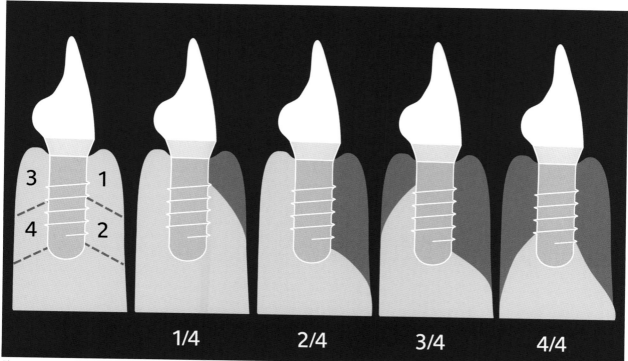

Fig 39 *Classification of alveolar bone defects by Terheyden (2010), defining the typical pattern of resorption that an alveolar crest will undergo in the wake of tooth extraction. Defect types are grouped into four quarters that relate the amount of existing bone loss to the position of a prospective dental implant. In the initial phase of resorption, the facial bone plate is reduced to less than 50% of the prospective implant length; defects of this type in single-tooth edentulous spaces are typically contained and are referred to as dehiscence defects when an implant is already present (1/4). Continued buccal resorption will then create a knife-edge narrow ridge that is not yet reduced in height while showing a buccal reduced to more than 50% of the prospective implant length (2/4). It will normally take years for tooth loss to result in partial (3/4) and finally complete (4/4) height reduction of the ridge via resorption of its oral component.*

Table 1 Overview of ridge defects.

Defect type	Single-tooth gap	Extended edentulous space, free-end situation	Completely edentulous jaw
1/4	Dehiscence defect, self-containing	Multiple dehiscence defects, self-containing	Multiple dehiscence defects, self-containing
2/4	Horizontal defect, non-self-containing, requires a ugmentation outside of the existing bony envelope	Horizontal defect, non-self-containing, requires augmentation outside of the existing bony envelope	Knife-edge ridge
3/4	Combined horizontal and vertical defect	Combined horizontal and vertical defect	Vertically reduced knife-edge ridge (Cawood class IV)
4/4	Through-and-through defect	Strictly vertical defect	Total jaw atrophy (Cawood classes V and VI)

Table 2   Preferred and alternative techniques for defects related to single missing teeth.

Defect classification Single-tooth gap	Description	Preferred technique	Alternative techniques	
1/4	Self-containing dehiscence defect with bone eminences next to the adjacent teeth	GBR simultaneously with implant placement	Staged GBR, simultaneous or staged bone block in the esthetic zone	
2/4	Non-self-containing horizontal defect requiring augmentation outside of the existing bony envelope	Staged GBR	GBR simultaneously with implant placement	In the esthetic zone: staged bone block
3/4	Combined horizontal and vertical defect	Staged GBR combined with a space-preserving device	Bone block, shell technique	
4/4	Through-and-through defect	Staged bone block	Staged GBR with a space-preserving device	

Table 3   *Preferred and alternative techniques defects related to extended edentulous spaces.*

Defect classification Extended edentulous space	Description	Preferred technique	Alternative techniques	
1/4	Self-containing horizontal defect	Staged GBR	GBR simultaneously with implant placement	In the esthetic zone: bone block, staged or simultaneously with implant placement
2/4	Non-self-containing horizontal defect requiring augmentation outside of the existing bony envelope	Less than 4 mm: staged bone block	Greater than 4 mm: ridge splitting	GBR, staged or simultaneously with implant placement
3/4	Combined horizontal and vertical defect	Bone block, shell technique	Staged GBR with space-preserving device	Swinging interpositional graft
4/4	Strictly vertical defect	Interpositional graft, sandwich technique	Staged onlay block	Distraction osteogenesis

Table 4   *Preferred and alternative techniques for defects related to edentulous jaws.*

Defect classification Edentulous jaw	Description	Preferred technique	Alternative techniques	
1/4	Multiple dehiscence defect	GBR simultaneously with implant placement	Staged GBR	In the esthetic zone: bone block simultaneously with implant placement
2/4	Knife-edge ridge	Staged bone blocks either from the ramus or an extraoral donor site	Greater than 4 mm: ridge splitting	
3/4	Vertically reduced knife-edge ridge (Cawood class IV)	For overdentures: Height reduction and short implants	For fixed restorations in the maxilla: Le Fort I interpositional graft	Bone block from the ramus or an extraoral donor site
4/4	Total jaw atrophy (Cawood classes V and VI)	Maxilla		
		Le Fort I interpositional graft from extraoral sites	Bone-block onlay graft	
		Mandible		
		For overdentures: no augmentation and short implants	For fixed restorations: interpositional grafting	In case of pending fracture: bone-block onlay graft

4.15 Wound Infection Prophylaxis and Antibiotics

Any surgical intervention inside the oral cavity will carry an increased risk of infection compared to procedures that are conducted through the external skin. Intraoral wounds will inevitably become contaminated with bacteria. Depending on the nature of a procedure, an infection rate of roughly 5% is common in implant dentistry (Tan and coworkers 2013; Esposito and coworkers 2010; Barone and coworkers 2006). It is mandatory to communicate this risk to patients beforehand and to obtain their informed consent.

Four steps are required to prevent bacterial infection during implant treatments that involve bone grafts (Table 5). The first step is to manage dental pathologies (e.g. by removing caries and by periodontal treatment) before proceeding to elective surgery. The second step is to implement professional tooth cleaning a few days

or immediately before surgery. Next, the patient should undertake a disinfecting mouth rinse preoperatively to reduce bacterial concentrations inside the oral cavity and the bacterial load of the surgical wound. In the fourth step, the patient should receive perioperative antibiotics. Beta-lactam-resistant amoxicillin is the drug of choice; clindamycin is a viable alternative in patients allergic to penicillins. Whether the antibiotic prescription should be extended over several days after the intervention remains open to debate. This decision is up to the clinician's judgment and needs to be made on a case-by-case basis. Possible side effects of long-term broad-spectrum antibiotics on the intestinal flora, including diarrhea and potentially lifethreatening pseudomembranous colitis, should be taken into account. There is preliminary evidence that probiotics may avoid complications of this type (Johnston and coworkers 2012).

Table 5   Stair concept with four steps of infection prophylaxis. Oral hygiene should be performed carefully by the patient after surgery, beginning on the first postoperative day. Tooth brushing is encouraged in the oral regions not involved in surgery, while chlorhexidine mouth rinses are prescribed twice daily.

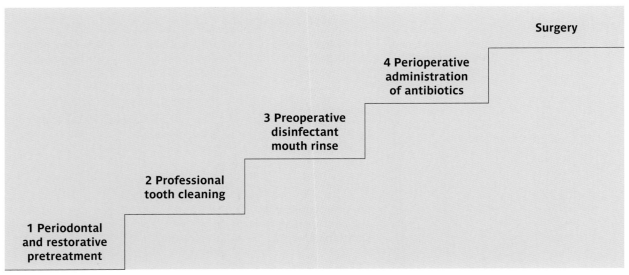

4.16 Medications and Postoperative Care

Conscious sedation is recommended for major augmentation procedures under local anesthesia, midazolam being the drug of choice. Some procedures like major iliac-crest harvesting or Le Fort I osteotomies will require general anesthesia.

Corticosteroids have a proven beneficial effect on postoperative sequelae such as trismus, swelling, and pain in cases of third-molar surgery, and a similar effect can be postulated for systemic steroids in cases of implant surgery.

Intraoral dressings are not required for augmentation procedures. Extraorally applied ice packs may help to reduce swelling. Patients should preferably take a seated position at rest and, during the first postoperative night, may lie down with the upper part of the body slightly raised. Analgesics are usually required for some days after surgery.

The sutures are removed after 10 days. No further medication or special care is needed after suture removal. Osteoporotic patients in particular should reduce their biting function for 6 weeks to avoid a risk of mandibular fracture.

4.17 Provisional Prostheses

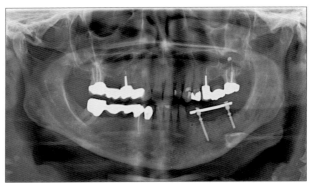

Fig 40a   Panoramic radiograph. Provisional restoration implemented as a fixed partial denture (FPD) made from resin with a metal wire for reinforcement.

It is important to avoid any mechanical loading of augmented areas. Removable partial dentures supported by the mucosa are contraindicated following augmentation surgery. If neighboring teeth are present, it is better to use a tooth-supported provisional solution. In the absence of neighboring teeth temporary implants may be used to support a removable prosthesis (Figs 40a-c, 41a-e, and 42a-d) or alternatively, no provisional prosthesis in the initial healing phase may be recommended.

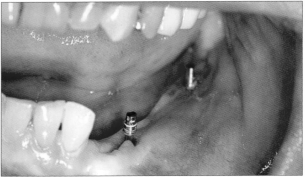

Fig 40b   Situation after placing the two temporary implants.

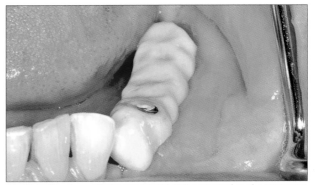

Fig 40c   Situation with the provisional FPD cemented to the temporary implants.

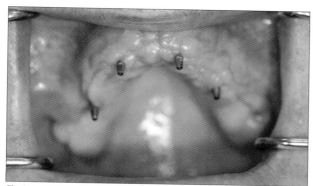

Fig 41a Temporary implants have been placed during tooth extraction to transition the patient from a dentate state to an implant-supported prosthesis. Moderate chewing is possible.

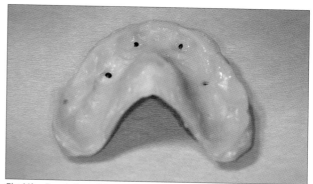

Fig 41b Basal view of the provisional overdenture.

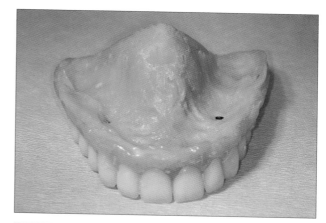

Fig 41c Frontal view of the provisional overdenture.

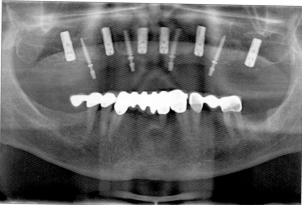

Fig 41d Panoramic radiograph obtained 3 months after tooth extraction. At this time, surgery for bone augmentation and placement of the definitive implants is performed. The provisional implants had been placed between the definitive implants as guided by the setup and drill template.

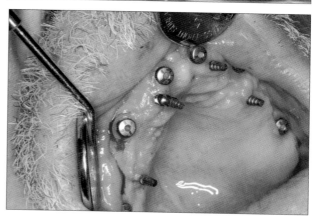

Fig 41e The provisional implants are removed during the re-entry surgery for implant exposure. A more buccal position of the definitive implants is noted following augmentation, demonstrating the effectiveness of buccal horizontal grafting.

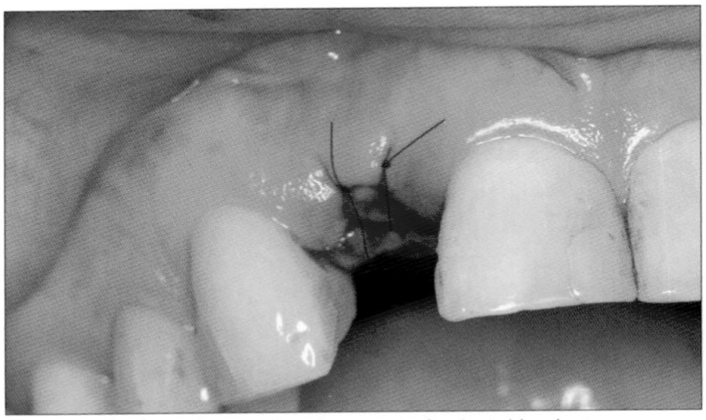

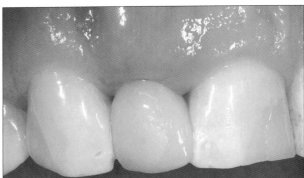

Fig 42a   Single-tooth gap after placement of a dental implant.

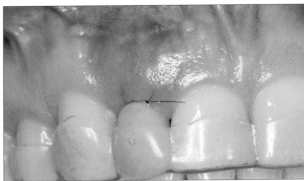

Fig 42b   An Essex retainer is used to provide a pontic designed to shape and support the soft tissues. This structure offers the advantage of being removable to access the wound within the first 2 postoperative weeks.

Fig 42c   After uneventful healing, the removable pontic is replaced by a fixed pontic bonded with resin to the neighboring teeth. This pontic will support the papillae.

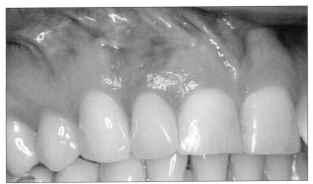

Fig 42d   Final restoration with ideal configuration of the peri-implant soft tissue.

5 <u>Implant Placement in Augmented Sites and Treatment Outcomes</u>

H. Terheyden, L. Cordaro

5.1 Implant Placement in Augmented Sites

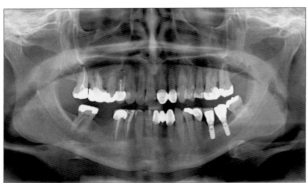

Fig 1a 3/4 defect at site 46 (combined horizontal and vertical bone defect).

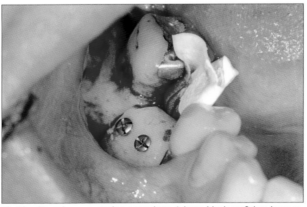

Fig 1b Staged augmentation procedure. A bone-block graft has been secured with two mini-lag screws (Twin Box 1.5 mm; Synthes, Tuttlingen, Germany), and a resorbable collagen membrane (Bio-Gide; Geistlich, Wolhusen, Switzerland) is already in place. Particulate autologous bone from a bone trap will be added underneath the membrane.

5.1.1 Healing Time of Bone-Block and GBR Reconstructions

An important consideration in staged procedures of bone augmentation is how much time should elapse between the reconstruction and implant stages. This interval should be long enough to allow the graft to become incorporated into the recipient site and for vital bone to form in the reconstructed ridge. It takes some time for a graft to heal, but the precise duration may vary with the nature of the graft, the grafting technique and, if applicable, the type of membrane used. Various authors using different techniques have reported intervals of 3 to 12 months from reconstruction to implant placement (Jensen and Terheyden 2009).

Onlay bone blocks will usually undergo significant surface resorption if the waiting period is longer than 4 to 6 months. Second-stage surgery performed later than this may disclose this resorption by screw heads protruding from the bone surface upon flap elevation. Nor is a waiting period shorter than 4 months advisable, since this carries a risk of dislodging the block from the underlying bone surface during implant installation. Local differences in bone hardness and graft maturation may result in technical difficulties during implant placement (Figs 1a-i).

A longer healing period of 9 to 12 months is usually required for large reconstructions of the GBR type with bone substitute materials (Jensen and Terheyden 2009). From a clinical point of view, GBR techniques may avoid donor-site surgery but will increase treatment durations.

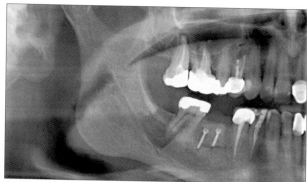

Fig 1c   Successful outcome of vertical and horizontal augmentation. The defect on the apical and distal aspects of tooth 37 is due to bone harvesting.

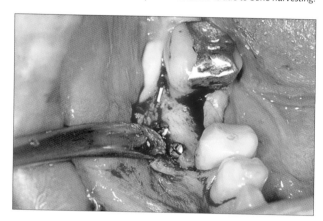

Fig 1d   Re-entry procedure after 4 months of healing. A full-thickness flap has been reflected. Note how the screw heads slightly protrude from the bone surface compared to Figure 1b. This discrepancy is due to surface resorption of the bone graft. A waiting period of less than 4 to 6 months would not have ensured adequate stability and integration of the graft, while a longer interval would have increasingly resulted in loss of graft volume.

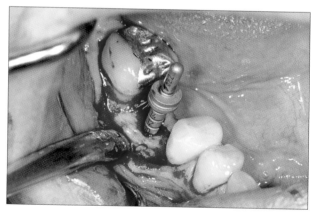

Fig 1e   Positioning an implant in grafted bone may be clinically difficult due to the difference in hardness between the graft from the linea obliqua and the preexisting alveolar bone. There is a need to consider these differences beforehand during preparation of the implant bed because they carry a risk of displacing the implant drill. Frequent use of the implant positioning aid is recommended.

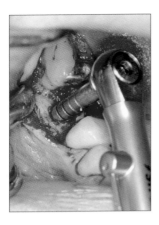

Fig 1f   Another problem of implant placement in grafted bone is the hardness of the bone-block graft. Pre-tapping of the threads was required in this case to reduce the insertion torque of the implant.

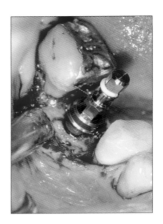

Fig 1g   An implant (Standard Plus TL WN, diameter 4.8 mm; Straumann, Basel, Switzerland) was placed and scheduled for transgingival healing. If a transmucosal protocol is used in this kind of situation, the bone-block graft will be in contact with the bacterially contaminated oral cavity, possibly resulting in secondary graft infection unless the bone block is completely integrated by the time of implant placement. For this reason, a submerged healing protocol using bone-level implants should be considered.

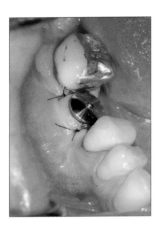

Fig 1h   The residual gingiva has adapted nicely to the healing abutment. No scars are visible. To achieve this kind of outcome, a midcrestal incision and a full-thickness flap should be used throughout all surgical steps.

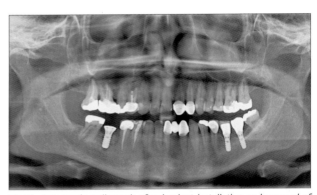

Fig 1i   Panoramic radiograph after implant installation and removal of the bone fixation screws.

5.1.2 Re-entry Stage and Removal of Osteosynthesis Materials

The authors recommend that all metal devices used for bone fixation in ridge augmentation procedures should be removed prior to implant placement. While these materials are usually made from titanium and cause no foreign-body or any other adverse reactions, they may interfere with implant-bed preparation and may become exposed as remodeling of the graft continues or if peri-implant bone loss develops. Any lag screws that were used to fixate a block graft can normally be removed quite easily, reducing trauma to the patient and limiting the duration of surgery. Screws in block grafts are removed on reopening the flap 4 months after the augmentation procedure at the time of implant placement. However, since reflection of a full-thickness flap will cause the bone to undergo some surface resorption, the surgeon will normally want to avoid broad exposure (unless required for implant placement) notably in the esthetic zone. The screws may be removed via multiple tiny stab incisions just above the screw heads visible/palpable under the soft tissue.

In GBR cases, too, the first measure during the second surgical stage will be to remove any materials like non-resorbable membranes, titanium mesh, or plates and screws that may have served to protect a particulate graft. While the grafted site needs to be extensively exposed in these situations, minimal flap reflection may be adequate for implant placement if a resorbable membrane—which does not need to be removed—was used.

Different techniques and hardware elements are eligible for implant placement, including either one-piece or two-piece implants left to heal either transmucosally or submerged. Recent studies have yielded no difference between bone-level (two-piece) and tissue-level implants following staged procedures with autologous bone grafting (Chiapasco and coworkers 2012a, Chiapasco and coworkers 2012b).

At esthetic sites, the ITI generally recommends that clinicians follow a submerged or semi-submerged protocol even if a ridge reconstruction has preceded implant placement by several months.

In considering implant types after staged ridge reconstruction, clinicians should always select a system that is well documented, has been scientifically validated, and is known to involve a low rate of marginal bone resorption.

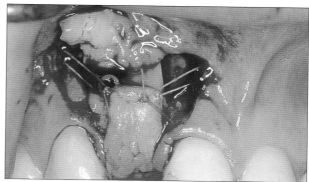

Fig 2a   Complex bone-block reconstruction of a lateral incisor site after previous implant loss. A titanium screw (Center Drive 2.0 mm; Martin, Tuttlingen, Germany) is used for fixation and a vascularized connective-tissue flap from the palate for coverage of the graft and the simultaneous dental implant.

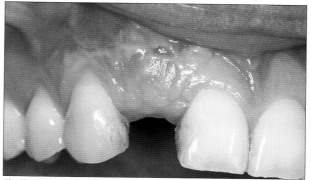

Fig 2b   Clinical situation after 4 months of healing. The head of the titanium screw is palpable under the mucosa and visible as a grayish shade.

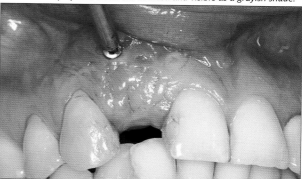

Fig 2c   Complete flap reflection to remove the screw would induce surface resorption and jeopardize the augmentative outcome. Instead, the screw is removed by exploring its head through a tiny stab incision for subsequent engagement of the screwdriver.

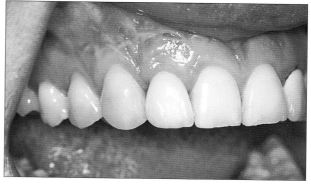

Fig 2d   Esthetic outcome.

5.2   Treatment Outcomes after Implant Placement

5.2.1   Implant Survival

A systematic review by Jensen and Terheyden (2009) on localized ridge defects in partially edentulous patients was presented at the 4th ITI Consensus Conference in 2008. The results showed a documented median survival of 100% (range: 96.9%–100%) for implants that had been placed in staged procedures following horizontal ridge augmentation 12 to 60 months after loading. Likewise, a median survival rate of 100% (range 95%–100%) was also identified for implants placed in staged procedures with vertical ridge augmentation. While it was not possible to relate implant survival to specific augmentation materials or methods based on the available data, it was possible to conclude that augmented bone did not differ from non-augmented native bone in terms of implant survival.

A second systematic review, presented by Chiapasco and coworkers (2009), was devoted to major defects in completely edentulous ridges. Its results showed a documented mean survival of 87% (95% in the mandible and 82% in the maxilla) for implants associated with onlay grafts. Le Fort I interpositional grafting of the maxilla was found to involve a 88% rate of implant survival overall, although this rate was up to 93% when only studies of implants featuring a roughened surface were considered. Distraction osteogenesis for vertical ridge augmentation was associated with an implant survival rate of 96.9%. Four studies could be included to evaluate ridge splitting with immediate implant placement, which yielded a median survival rate of 94%. No studies or data were available for staged ridge splitting.

Aghaloo and Moy (2007) published a meta-analysis of materials and methods for alveolar bone augmentation. They identified a mean survival rate of 95.5% (confidence interval: 92%–99%) for implants placed in staged procedures with vertical and horizontal GBR. Two reports on ridge splitting that involved a relatively great number of implants yielded a mean survival rate

of 97.4%. Onlay and veneer grafting with autologous bone blocks was reported to yield a mean survival rate of 90.4%, and implants placed in conjunction with interpositional grafts survived in 83.8% of cases. The authors did point out, however, that the reviewed studies were highly heterogeneous and covered dissimilar baseline situations ranging from local defects to edentulous jaws. Hence the outcomes of their review should be interpreted with caution.

Esposito and coworkers (2010) published a Cochrane review of comparative studies dealing with different augmentation techniques and materials. They arrived at an odds ratio of 5.74 (CI: 0.92–35.82) for implant failure on comparing results for short implants associated with vertical augmentation, although this findings was based on only two studies.

5.2.2   Augmentative Effects of Different Materials and Techniques

The systematic review by Jensen and Terheyden (2009) yielded a mean gain in bone width of 3.6 mm for staged procedures of horizontal augmentation, with 11.1% of cases requiring additional grafting at the time of re-entry. Non-resorbable membranes for staged horizontal augmentation yielded a mean gain of 2.9 mm and additional grafting requirements in 19.8% of cases. The corresponding figures for resorbable membranes were 4.2 mm and 4.1%, respectively. In the absence of a membrane, 4.5 mm were gained and 13.9% required additional grafting. Space-preserving autologous blocks for horizontal grafting yielded a mean gain of 4.4 mm and additional grafting requirements in 2.8% of cases. In the absence of a bone block, the corresponding figures were 2.6 mm and 24.4%, respectively. Procedures of vertical augmentation yielded a mean gain in ridge height of 4.8 mm, with 26.4% of cases requiring additional grafting at re-entry. Mean gains of 3.5 versus 4.2 mm with additional grafting requirements in 32.8% versus 20% of cases were obtained in the presence or absence of a membrane, respectively. Autologous block grafts versus particulate materials for staged vertical augmentation were associated with gains of 3.7 versus 3.6 mm and additional grafting requirements in 16.9% versus 32.6% of cases.

In their Cochrane review, Esposito and coworkers (2010) identified no significant differences between horizontal augmentation techniques based on three included trials. Eight included trials dealing with vertical bone augmentation, for the most part, again did not show significant differences between techniques. Three of them did reveal more pronounced vertical gains by osteodistraction than with autologous inlay grafts (mean difference: 3.25 mm; 95% CI: 1.66 – 4.84) and by using a bone substitute rather than autologous bone for GBR (mean difference 0.60 mm; 95% CI 0.21 – 0.99) in atrophic posterior mandibles. Patients were found to favor a bone substitute over autologous bone harvested from the iliac crest (OR = 0.03; 95% CI: 0.00 – 0.64; p = 0.02).

5.2.3 Complication Rates of Different Materials and Techniques

The systematic review by Jensen and Terheyden (2009) revealed a mean complication rate of 12.2% for staged procedures of horizontal augmentation. The use of non-resorbable versus resorbable membranes was as-sociated with mean complication rates of 23.6% versus 18.9%; in the absence of a membrane, the rate was 9.4%. The use of space-preserving autologous blocks was associated with a mean complication rate of 3.8%; in the absence of a bone block, the rate was 39.6%. Vertical augmentation procedures were found to involve premature exposure of grafting materials in 18.8% of cases. Mean complication rates of 23.2% or 25.3% were associated with the presence or absence of a membrane, respectively, and autologous block grafts versus particulate materials for staged vertical augmentation were found to involve complication rates of 29.8% versus 21.0%.

Chiapasco and coworkers (2009), in their systematic review on augmentation techniques for major defects in completely edentulous ridges, calculated a complication rate of 4.7% for onlay grafts while pointing out that healed onlay grafts from the iliac crest were affected by resorption at high rates of 12% to 60% over 5 years. Distraction osteogenesis involved a mean complication rate of 27% and Le Fort I interpositional grafting a mean rate of 3.1% in that review. Iliac-crest harvesting was associated with protracted pain and gait disturbances in 2% of cases. By comparison, the rate of protracted pain after calvarial harvesting was 0%.

In their Cochrane review, Esposito and coworkers (2010) arrived at an odds ratio of 4.97 (95% CI: 1.1 – 22.4) for complications comparing vertical augmentations with short implants, although this finding was based on only two studies.

6   Clinical Case Presentations

6.1   Autologous Block Graft and Guided Bone Regeneration (GBR) for Horizontal Ridge Augmentation in the Anterior Maxilla

D. Buser, U. Belser

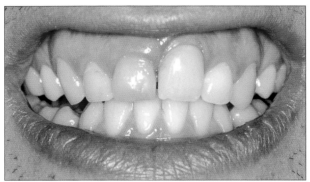

Fig 1   Clinical view of a demanding initial situation. A high smile line and gingival recession at tooth 21.

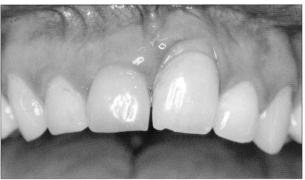

Fig 2   Close-up view of the apically malpositioned and ankylosed tooth 21. The situation is associated with significant gingival recession. In addition, tooth 11 is non-vital and requires treatment to eliminate or mask its discoloration.

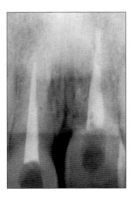

Fig 3   Periapical radiographs. Both teeth (11 and 21) had previously undergone root-canal treatment but were not afflicted by apical pathology. Root 21 exhibits typical signs of ankylosis and external root resorption.

A 27-year-old man was referred to the Department of Oral Surgery and Stomatology (University of Bern, Switzerland) for implant therapy in the anterior maxilla. The patient was healthy and did not smoke. His tooth 21 was apically malpositioned and ankylosed due to a dental trauma during adolescence. The preoperative examination included an esthetic risk assessment (Martin and coworkers 2006), which revealed a number of high-risk factors, most important among them the patient's high smile line and the non-harmonious gingival margins of the maxillary anterior dentition (Fig 1). Tooth 21 was associated with significant gingival recession (Fig 2). Tooth 11 required treatment to eliminate or mask severe discoloration from previous root canal treatment. A periapical radiograph confirmed the ankylosed condition of root 21 and disclosed characteristic signs of advanced external root resorption, also showing that both central incisors had been exposed to root canal treatment. Neither tooth showed signs of apical pathology (Fig 3).

After discussing the situation with the patient, it was agreed to proceed with the following treatment plan:

- Extraction of the ankylosed central incisor with a minor flap elevation and primary soft-tissue closure to correct the soft-tissue deficiency
- Attempt at non-vital bleaching of tooth 11
- Horizontal ridge augmentation of site 21 using an autologous block graft and GBR
- Six months later, implant placement into the augmented ridge at site 21
- Delivery of implant-supported single crown at site 21 and a ceramic veneer at tooth 11 (unless the tooth would respond to non-vital bleaching)

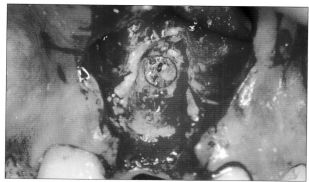

Fig 4 Clinical status after removing the ankylosed root 21. A through-and-through bone defect was present at the palatal aspect.

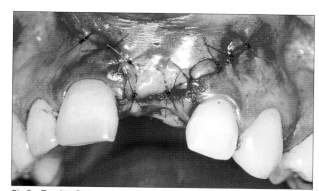

Fig 5 Tension-free wound closure after performing a periosteal incision.

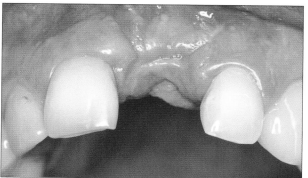

Fig 6 Soft-tissue healing was uneventful. The future implant site 21 was associated with an adequate band of keratinized mucosa.

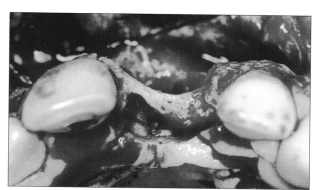

Fig 7 This occlusal view was obtained during the second surgical session and reveals a flattened bone defect with a crest width of only 3 mm at site 21.

As expected, it was quite difficult to remove the ankylosed tooth 21. The root could not be mobilized on elevating a small trapezoidal mucoperiosteal flap via papilla-sparing vertical incisions, and it therefore had to be removed in small pieces following longitudinal root splitting. Finally, a large round diamond bur was used to eliminate all remnants of the ankylosed root.

A small bone defect extended to the palatal aspect of the alveolar crest (Fig 4). Surgical exposure confirmed the presence of a large flattened bone defect, which required a second surgical procedure for horizontal ridge augmentation, allowing for correct placement of an implant in a third surgery. The surgical tooth removal included an incision of the periosteum and tension-free primary wound closure to eliminate the vertical soft-tissue deficiency (Fig 5). Good progress of soft-tissue healing was noted after some weeks (Fig 6).

Around 2 months later, the second procedure was conducted under local anesthesia with sedative premedication. Site 21 was exposed by raising a trapezoidal mucoperiosteal flap and using vertical releasing incisions at both adjacent teeth (this was the standard flap technique used by our group for single-tooth replacements in 2001, when this patient was treated).

As expected, a large flattened bone defect was present on the facial aspect of site 21. The remaining crest width of 3 mm (Fig 7) was too narrow to allow for implant placement with simultaneous contour augmentation by GBR. The anticipated staged approach of initially using an autologous block graft for horizontal augmentation along with GBR was therefore adopted.

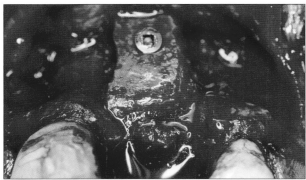

Fig 8   Ridge augmentation was initiated with a corticocancellous block graft harvested from the chin. The graft was stabilized with a self-tapping miniscrew to ensure stability of the wound in the augmented region.

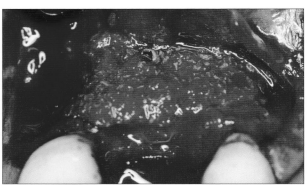

Fig 9   Autologous bone chips were used to fill voids around the block graft. The entire area was covered with DBBM particles to establish a continuous convex profile.

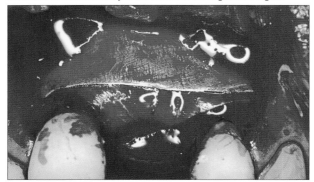

Fig 10   The augmentation material was covered with a double layer of resorbable collagen membrane as a temporary barrier against ingrowth of soft-tissue cells during the initial phase of wound healing.

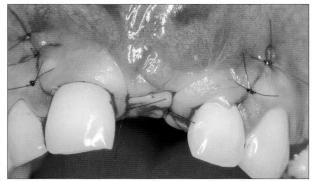

Fig 11   Surgery was finalized by tension-free primary wound closure, which required an incision of the periosteum to mobilize the flap.

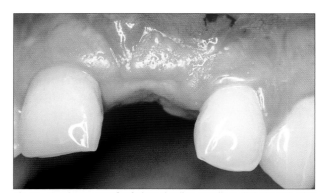

Fig 12   Good progress of soft-tissue healing. Excellent clinical result after 5 months.

A block graft 16 × 9 × 5 mm in size was harvested from the chin area. Before applying it to the future implant site, the cortical bone surface was perforated with a small round bur to open the marrow cavity of the recipient site. The block graft was applied with its cancellous portion facing the bleeding bone surface and stabilized with a self-tapping miniscrew (Fig 8).

All lateral voids were filled by applying small autologous bone chips to the block. Subsequent addition of a thin superficial layer of DBBM (deproteinized bovine bone mineral) available as Bio-Oss® (Geistlich Biomaterials, Wolhusen, Switzerland) resulted in a theoretical crest width of about 8 mm (Fig 9).

A resorbable collagen membrane (Bio-Gide®; Geistlich Biomaterials) was used to cover the grafting material (Fig 10). Surgery was finalized by tension-free primary wound closure with 4-0 and 5-0 monofilament polyamide suture material (Fig 11). Postsurgical wound healing was uneventful and resulted in well-matured mucosa.

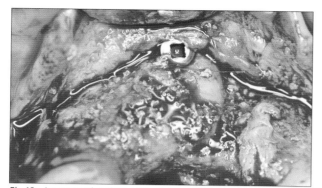

Fig 13   Intraoperative views of the third surgical session. The position of the miniscrew indicated that the block graft had undergone minimal resorption.

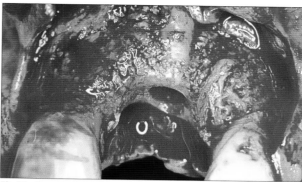

Fig 14   It was not possible to fully compensate for the vertical bone deficiency.

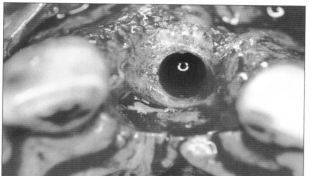

Fig 15   Given the new crest width of roughly 8 mm, a screw-type titanium implant offering a diameter of 4 mm could be placed.

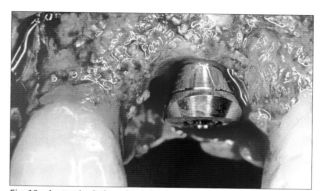

Fig 16   A standard tissue-level implant was selected whose shoulder was positioned around 2 mm apical to the facial mucosal margin of the planned implant-supported crown. A beveled healing cap was attached to the implant.

After 6 months of healing, the site was reopened for the third surgical session, this time to insert an implant into the augmented ridge. The flap elevated for this purpose revealed a well-healed edentulous ridge and an excellent regenerative outcome. The block graft was well integrated and—as indicated by the position of the fixation screw head—had not undergone superficial resorption (Figs 13 and 14).

Given the new crest width of 8 mm, a tissue-level implant with a diameter of 4.1 mm (Straumann, Basel, Switzerland) could be placed (Figs 15 and 16). After attaching a beveled healing cap, primary wound closure was achieved for submerged wound healing (Fig 17).

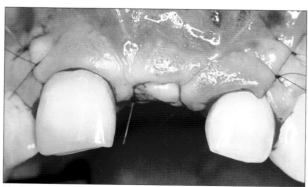

Fig 17   Submerged healing achieved by primary wound closure.

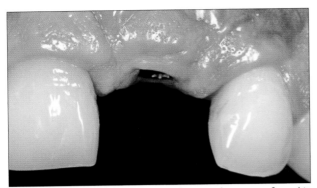

Fig 18   At 8 weeks, a punch-type reopening procedure was performed to gain access to the implant.

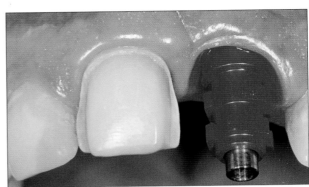

Fig 19   Prior to taking an open-tray impression of the implant shoulder at site 21 in the presence of a screw-retained impression coping, the severely discolored tooth 11 had been prepared for a laminate ceramic veneer.

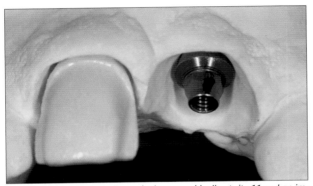

Fig 20   Master cast including a single removable die at site 11 and an implant analog at site 21, to which a long synOcta abutment was connected for direct establishment of the screw connection with the restoration.

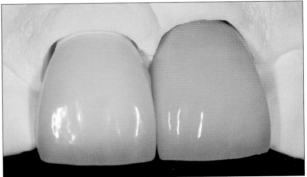

Fig 21   Close-up view of the two completed ceramic restorations, one a laminate veneer on a natural tooth (site 11), the other one an implant-supported crown (site 21).

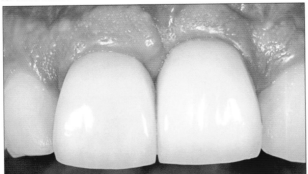

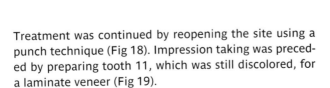

Fig 22   Clinical views of the anterior maxilla shortly after insertion of the two ceramic restorations. Newly established symmetry both of the relative tooth dimensions and of the mucosal line.

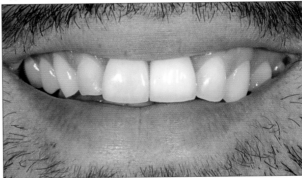

Fig 23   View of the patient's non-forced smile. Harmony of restorative integration had been achieved.

Treatment was continued by reopening the site using a punch technique (Fig 18). Impression taking was preceded by preparing tooth 11, which was still discolored, for a laminate veneer (Fig 19).

A revision of the root-canal treatment had been carried out previously and was followed by an unsuccessful bleaching attempt. The resultant master cast featured both a retrievable die at site 11 and an implant analog supporting a synOcta abutment at site 21 (Fig 20).

Restorative therapy included a screw-retained metal-ceramic crown on the implant and a ceramic veneer masking the discoloration of tooth 11 (Fig 21). The esthetic outcome was quite pleasing, not least because the initially pronounced soft-tissue recession at site 21 had been nearly eliminated.

Clinical views reveal adequate esthetics with symmetrical tissue volumes (Figs 22 and 23). The periapical radiograph confirms that the tissue-level implant was well integrated after treatment (Fig 24).

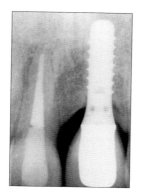

Fig 24 Periapical radiograph. Good integration of the tissue-level implant.

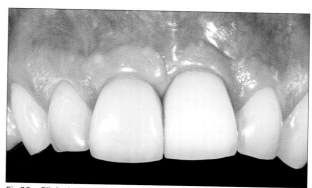

Fig 25 Clinical status at the 10-year follow-up. The peri-implant soft tissue was healthy and stable, except for minor soft-tissue recession at tooth 11.

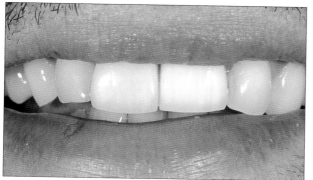

Fig 26 The overall esthetic outcome was very pleasing at the 10-year follow-up.

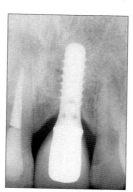

Fig 27 Periapical radiograph obtained at the 10-year follow-up. Excellent stability of the crestal bone levels.

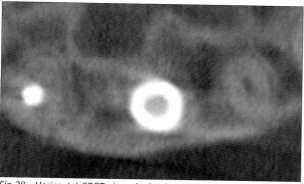

Fig 28 Horizontal CBCT view obtained at the 10-year follow-up. Intact facial bone wall.

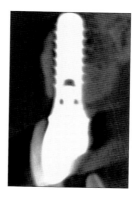

Fig 29 Orofacial CBCT view. The facial bone wall was fully intact and 1 to 1.5 mm thick.

The patient was scheduled for an aftercare maintenance program. His compliance remained consistently good both in terms of self-performed hygiene and in returning for the periodic recalls. At the 10-year follow-up, his clinical status was characterized by good mucosal health and stability at the implant-supported crown. Mild gingival recession was noted at the natural tooth 11, where the margin of the ceramic veneer was visible. A minor step apparent at the incisal edge indicated that some growth had taken place in the alveolar crest during the 10 years of implant function (Figs 25 and 26).

A periapical radiograph at the 10-year follow-up revealed stable levels of the peri-implant bone crest (Fig 27). An additional CBCT scan (4 × 4 cm) confirmed the presence of an intact facial bone wall (around 1.5 mm thick) at the implant site (Figs 28 and 29).

Discussion

Guided bone regeneration (GBR) is a well-documented treatment option for horizontal ridge augmentation. It was developed in the late 1980s after promising results had been obtained in preclinical studies (Dahlin and coworkers 1988; Dahlin and coworkers 1989; Dahlin and coworkers 1990). The first barrier membranes used in implant patients at the University of Bern (Switzerland) date back to October 1988; both the first case report and the first clinical study were published in 1990 (Nyman and coworkers 1990; Buser and coworkers 1990). Over the past 25 years, the GBR technique was gradually improved through modifications introduced to the surgical protocol and increasingly better biomaterials.

Today, the GBR technique is routinely used to regenerate local bone at implant sites, either simultaneously with implant placement or with a staged approach (Buser 2009). A simultaneous approach is preferred because it minimizes the number of surgical interventions and morbidity while also lowering cost. Simultaneous GBR is predominantly used for post-extraction implant placement, which has been covered extensively in Volume 3 of the ITI Treatment Guide series (Chen and Buser 2008). It may be used in peri-implant bone defects characterized with at least a two-wall morphology, which requires a crest width of at least 6 mm adjacent to the implant site (Buser 2009).

A staged approach is advisable for alveolar crests that show extensive flattening and are narrower than 4 mm in width. This was the situation in the present case. The staged approach includes a first surgical stage for horizontal ridge augmentation and a second stage for implant placement.

The earliest GBR procedures in implant dentistry were performed with non-resorbable membranes of the expanded polytetrafluoroethylene (ePTFE) type (Gore-Tex® Regenerative Membrane; W.L. Gore & Associates, Flagstaff, AZ, USA). In 1989, autologous block grafts were introduced to prevent these membranes from collapsing (Buser and coworkers 1990). This was followed by the introduction of stainless-steel miniscrews to stabilize the barrier membrane, an improvement to the surgical technique for horizontal augmentation published in a 1993 case report (Buser and coworkers 1993), followed by a case-series study of 40 consecutively treated patients (Buser and coworkers 1996). This latter study demonstrated highly predictable and good regenerative outcomes by combining autologous block grafts with a biologically inert non-resorbable ePTFE membrane and primary wound closure. Fairly small blocks were harvested for this application from either the chin or the retromolar region of the mandible. It turned out that those

blocks underwent almost no surface resorption during healing beneath the biologically inert membranes. Moreover, the related implants did well in terms of long-term stability, with a prospective study yielding a 5-year success rate of more than 98% (Buser and coworkers 2002).

However, this surgical technique was clinically demanding and carried an increased risk of complications in case a soft-tissue dehiscence occurred (Augthun and coworkers 1995). In the late 1990s, therefore, these limitations prompted efforts to simplify the surgical procedure and reduce the risk of complications. After a resorbable collagen membrane derived from porcine skin (Bio-Gide®; Geistlich Biomaterials, Wolhusen, Switzerland) had yielded promising results in a preclinical study (Hürzeler and coworkers 1998), it was decided to use this instead of the biologically inert non-resorbable e-PTFE membranes. This switch allowed for a less difficult surgical technique, since a collagen membrane did not require fixation with miniscrews due to its hydrophilic nature. A case-series study of 42 consecutive patients with the new membrane applied to 58 augmented sites (von Arx and Buser 2006) revealed both a greatly reduced risk of soft-tissue dehiscence and predictable amounts of horizontal bone gain (mean gain: 4.6 mm).

The patient case here presented was part of that prospective study. Despite the challenges posed by its initial clinical situation, an excellent long-term outcome has been achieved. The hardest part was to correct the vertical soft-tissue deficiency—significant in this case—often seen in posttraumatic situations with apically malpositioned and ankylosed teeth. The tooth had to be removed by minor flap elevation and root splitting, followed by tension-free soft-tissue closure after mobilizing the flap with a periosteal incision. An alternative would have been to shorten the root to 3 mm under the mucosal level and allowing spontaneous overgrowth, today a frequently used technique for treating apically malpositioned and ankylosed teeth as it offers an extra amount of keratinized mucosa (Langer 1994).

The use of corticocancellous block grafts has been known for predictable outcomes, as a block graft can be fixated with a miniscrew for good wound stabilization—stability of the grafted area is important for successful regenerative outcomes (von Arx and Buser 2009). It is also important to freshen the cortical bone surface of the recipient site to allow ingrowth of blood vessels into the coagulum and of new bone into the non-vital block graft (Burkhardt 1986). Such ingrowth appears to be essential to the long-term stability of these block grafts and has been referred to as "creeping substitution" to describe a mechanism in which necrotic bone of the block graft is gradually resorbed and replaced by new viable bone through the Haversian system (von Arx and coworkers 2001). Creeping substitution is only possible because of the presence of adequate nourishment from the recipient bed and structures surrounding the graft (Burkhardt and Enneking 1978).

The fact that an autologous block graft needs to be harvested is clearly a disadvantage of this surgical technique, considering that an extra surgical site adds to the duration of surgery, increases patient morbidity (von Arx and coworkers 2005), and increases cost. It might be possible to eliminate this drawback by switching to allogeneic or xenogeneic block grafts. Clinical studies are needed to demonstrate whether these alternative materials can replace autologous blocks for horizontal ridge augmentation by GBR in the near future.

Acknowledgment

The authors wish to thank Mr. Michel Magne, CDT and master ceramist, for his expertise and excellent fabrication of the ceramic restorations.

6.2 Staged GBR with Allogeneic Particulate Grafting Material for Single-Tooth Replacement

E. Lewis, F. Lozano

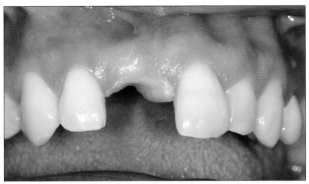

Fig 1 Frontal view of the single-tooth edentulous space at site 11.

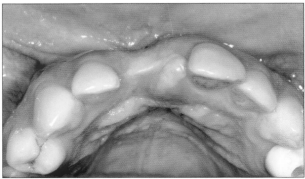

Fig 2 Occlusal view of the single-tooth edentulous space at site 11.

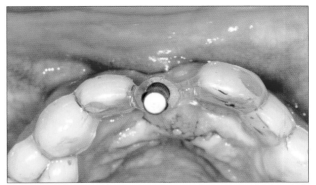

Fig 3 Pretreatment occlusal view with the surgical template in place, indicating the significant horizontal bone deficiency at site 11.

Staged bone augmentation of the alveolar ridge is indicated whenever a proposed implant site is deficient and will not support implant placement with simultaneous grafting. This is particularly true of healed sites presenting with facial flattening of the ridge. Since primary stability cannot possibly be achieved in this situation, it is recommended to use a staged approach with guided bone regeneration (GBR) for correct three-dimensional placement of the implant. In the anterior maxilla, staged GBR procedures are conducted not only to provide adequate bone volume for implant placement but also to restore a proper and stable contour of the orofacial ridge for improved long-term esthetics.

A case is presented that demonstrates the technique for single-tooth replacement utilizing a staged approach with a particulate grafting material.

A 50-year-old man whose tooth 11 was missing presented for consultation to the Center for Implant Dentistry in January 2010. He indicated that, having been provided with a resin removable partial denture after the tooth had been avulsed back in 1998, he now wanted to explore the option of fixed tooth replacement with a dental implant. The patient's medical history included well-controlled hypertension, and he was a non-smoker. High-profile public appearances related to his work accounted for his high esthetic expectations.

The clinical examination revealed a high smile line, good oral hygiene, and no evidence of periodontal disease. The missing tooth site 11 was associated with well-preserved papillae on the adjacent virgin teeth (Fig 1) but was significantly deficient horizontally (Figs 2 and 3). The patient stated that a midline diastema of around 1 mm had been present before the trauma.

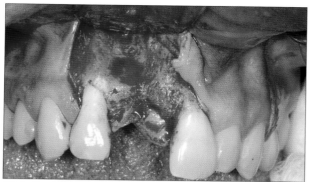

Fig 4 Frontal view of the bone defect after elevation of the mucoperiosteal flap.

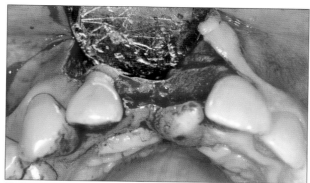

Fig 5 Occlusal view of the bone defect after elevation of the mucoperiosteal flap.

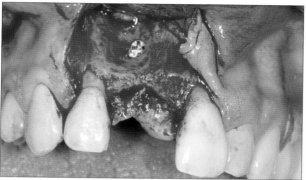

Fig 6 Frontal view of titanium tenting screw in place.

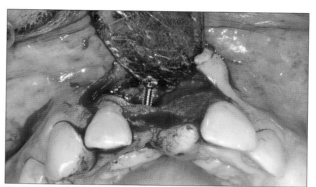

Fig 7 Occlusal view of titanium tenting screw in place.

A plain-film examination showed that bone height was adequate at site 11. No evidence of pathology was noted.

After discussing the procedure and grafting options, the patient elected to proceed with a treatment plan which included an implant-supported restoration preceded by bone augmentation (using an allogeneic particulate material of cadaveric origin) and which comprised the following four phases:

- Bone augmentation using a cadaveric particulate grafting material
- Implant placement following 6 months of healing and graft consolidation
- Implant provisionalization and soft-tissue contouring
- Recording of the soft-tissue contour and delivery of the final restoration

After the patient's consent had been obtained, the procedure was performed under local anesthesia on an outpatient basis. A two-sided incision was made, with a sulcular incision from the midfacial of tooth 21, extending across the edentulous crest to the distal aspect of tooth 12 with a vertical release. A full-thickness mucoperiosteal flap was elevated to expose the large facial deficiency at site 11 (Figs 4 and 5).

The defect was then thoroughly curetted free of soft tissue and irrigated with sterile saline. Periosteal release was performed to increase flap mobility. A titanium tenting screw (length: 9.0 mm; diameter: 1.5 mm) was placed into the central aspect of the defect at a 45° downward angle for ease of removal at the time of implant placement (Figs 6 and 7).

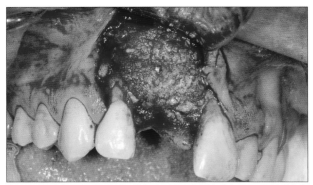

Fig 8 DFDBA packed into the defect around the tenting screw in a slightly overcontoured fashion.

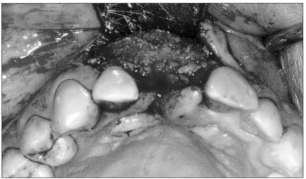

Fig 9 Occlusal view of DFDBA showing overcontoured augmentation.

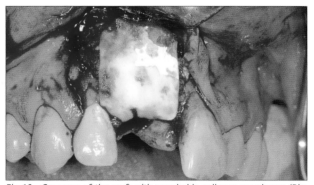

Fig 10 Coverage of the graft with resorbable collagen membrane (Bio-Gide; Geistlich Biomaterials, Wolhusen, Switzerland).

A block of demineralized freeze-dried bone allograft (DFDBA) (Regenaform®; Exactech, Gainsville, FL, USA) 1 cm³ in size was first placed into a warming bath (43–49 °C) for 5 minutes and was then transferred to the surgical site (Fig 8).

Using a curette and periosteal elevator, the allograft was gently packed around the tenting screw to augment the site in a slightly overcontoured fashion (Fig 9).

A resorbable collagen membrane (Bio-Gide; Geistlich Biomaterials, Wolhusen, Switzerland) 13 × 25 mm in size was then trimmed and placed over the facial aspect of the bone graft, tucking the inferior edge under the palatal edge of the mucosa (Fig 10).

Primary closure of the surgical site was achieved using 4-0 Vicryl™ (Ethicon, San Angelo, TX, USA) suture material (Figs 11 to 13).

Subsequently the removable partial denture was relieved to rule out pressure on the surgical site. The patient was given general postoperative instructions and prescriptions for a 1-week course of oral antibiotics (Amoxicillin 500 mg perorally three times a day), oral analgesics, and chlorhexidine digluconate 0.12% for rinsing. After 1 week, the surgical site was examined for incision closure and absence of infection. Postsurgical healing remained uneventful.

Following approximately 6 months of healing, the patient returned to the prosthodontist for diagnostic impressions to fabricate a surgical template.

The second phase of treatment consisted of implant placement. A two-stage approach was selected in order to maximize soft-tissue availability and aid in the wearing of the patient's removable partial denture. First, the template was placed in the patient's mouth to confirm its fit. The tissue was reflected to expose the healed graft site, and the titanium screw was removed. Using a restoration-driven surgical approach with a surgical template, a standard implant preparation was performed. After preparing the osteotomies in accordance with the manufacturer's instructions, a bone-level implant was placed at site 11 (Bone Level SLActive, diameter 4.1 mm, length 10 mm; Straumann, Basel, Switzerland). An internal healing cap was placed and primary wound closure achieved with 4-0 Vicryl™ sutures. The fit of the removable partial denture was checked and a periapical radiograph taken to confirm the implant position (Fig 14). Once again, healing was uneventful.

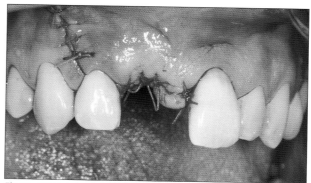

Fig 11   Frontal view after suturing.

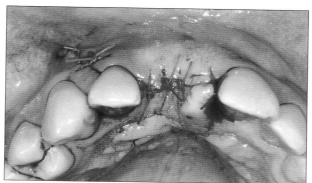

Fig 12   Occlusal view after suturing.

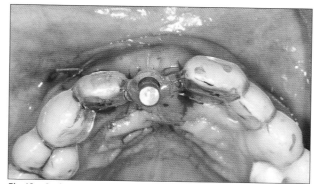

Fig 13   Occlusal view obtained with the template in place immediately after surgery, demonstrating the result of horizontal augmentation.

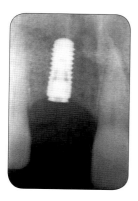

Fig 14   Periapical radiograph after implant placement.

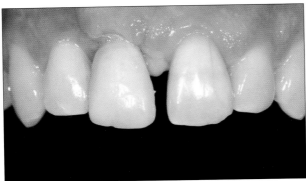

Fig 15   Frontal view of provisional restoration re-creating midline diastema.

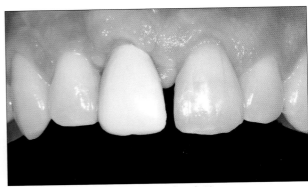

Fig 16   CAD/CAM full contour wax-up of tooth 11.

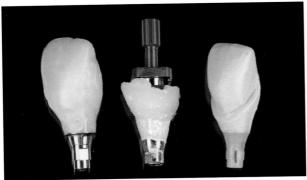

Fig 17   Provisional restoration on the left, custom impression post in the center, and wax-up cut back on the right.

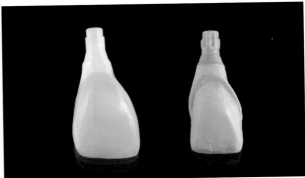

Fig 18   Final restoration and CAD/CAM wax-up that had been used in the laboratory to produce the final contours.

After the healing period, the patient returned for the next stage to have his implant uncovered, which was accomplished via a semilunar incision and rolling of a de-epithelialized pedicle in a facial direction under local anesthesia.

Later the patient returned to the prosthodontist for phases 3 and 4 of treatment. To this end, a provisional screw-retained restoration was fabricated on a titanium provisional cylinder (Fig 15). Tissue contouring was ac-complished in increments to maximize tissue support without causing excess recession on the midfacial as-pect. A customized impression post was utilized to re-cord the transition zone of the mucosa.

The full-contour wax-up was fabricated in CAD wax and tried in the mouth prior to scanning to verify final im-pression accuracy (Figs 16 to 18). The ceramist com-pleted the porcelain addition to the CAD/CAM Zirconia abutment to create a one-piece restoration.

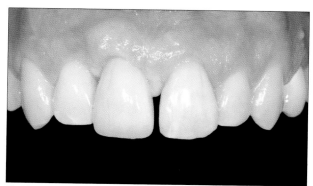

Fig 19   Frontal view of the final restoration in place.

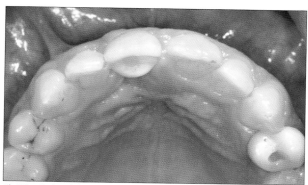

Fig 20   Occlusal view of the final restoration in place.

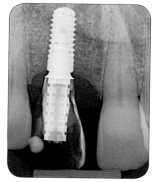

Fig 21   Periapical radiograph at the
time of loading.

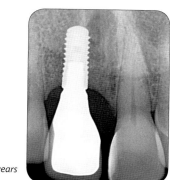

Fig 22   Periapical radiograph 2 years
after placement of implant 11.

The final implant-supported crown was adjusted and de-livered (Figs 19 and 20). The patient was pleased with the esthetic outcome and the improved confidence of having a fixed restoration.

Subsequently the patient entered the recall/mainte-nance phase of treatment and has recently attended his 2-year follow-up (Figs 21 to 23).

Acknowledgments

Ceramic laboratory procedures
M&M Dental Lab – Gainesville, FL, USA

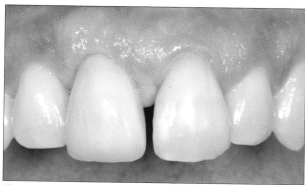

Fig 23   Frontal view at the 2-year follow-up.

6.3 Guided Bone Regeneration (GBR) with a Particulated Autologous Graft and an ePTFE-Reinforced Membrane for Vertical Augmentation of a Single-Tooth Edentulous Space in the Esthetic Zone

P. Casentini

A 47-year-old Caucasian woman with a single-tooth edentulous space at the site of the left maxillary canine was referred for treatment. She had undergone traumatic extraction of this impacted canine several months before referral. Her chief complaint was the dissatisfying appearance of her smile. The patient desired a stable and esthetic rehabilitation of the site. Her dental history showed no evidence of periodontal disease or bruxism. She had no systemic diseases, was not taking any medications, and did not smoke.

The extraoral examination revealed a high lip line and an inadequate soft-tissue volume at the defective canine site. Large black triangles were visible between the canine and its adjacent teeth (Fig 1).

Tooth 23 was missing and had been replaced with a temporary restoration bonded to the adjacent teeth. The profile of the alveolar process was reduced horizontally and vertically. While the adjacent teeth 22 and 24 showed some degree of soft-tissue recession with exposure of the cementoenamel junction, they were neither mobile nor associated with increased probing depths. Both the intermaxillary relationship and the interarch distance were normal (Fig 2).

Other than that, the state of the patient's remaining dentition was considered adequate. Her occlusion was normal and extended to the second molar. She exhibited healthy periodontal tissues with no signs of inflammation and no pathological probing.

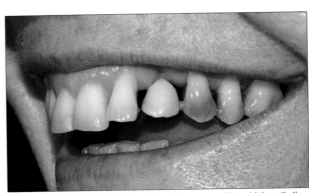

Fig 1   Initial situation with the existing defect exposed by a high smile line.

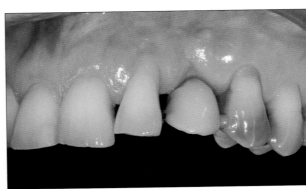

Fig 2   Intraoral view of the area.

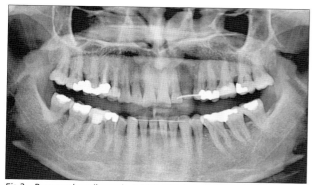

Fig 3   Panoramic radiograph. A wide defect at site 23.

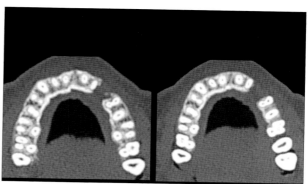

Fig 4   CT scan. Wall-to-wall defect at site 23.

While the patient's oral hygiene was also considered adequate, a minor modification of her brushing technique was suggested to avoid an increase in buccal recession. No pathology of the oral mucosa was diagnosed. The patient's esthetic expectations were realistic.

A preliminary panoramic radiograph revealed a large bone defect in association with reduced bone levels at the adjacent teeth (Fig 3). No significant alterations were noted in any other areas of the oral cavity. A computed-tomography (CT) scan confirmed the presence of a large defect with almost complete loss of both the buccal and palatal bone walls (Fig 4). The adjacent bone levels were to some extent preserved.

Treatment planning

Based on the clinical and radiological situation, the following treatment plan was proposed:

- An initial procedure of bone augmentation with autologous bone harvested from the oral cavity (mandibular ramus)
- Delayed placement of an implant at the site of the missing canine
- Temporary prosthetic restoration followed by definitive ceramic crowns (the first premolar had a large amalgam restoration and was included in the plan)

It was explained to the patient that the reduced bone levels at the sites adjacent to the missing canine made it unlikely that the soft tissue profile could be fully restored. She agreed to the treatment plan and gave her written informed consent.

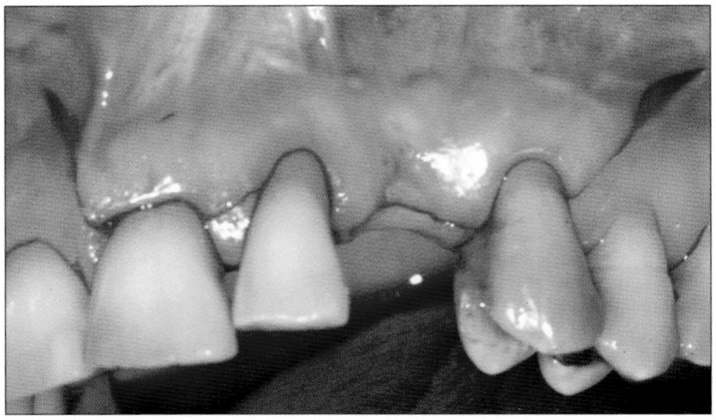

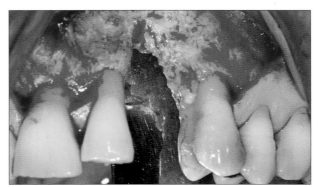

Fig 5   Flap design with releasing incisions at the adjacent teeth.

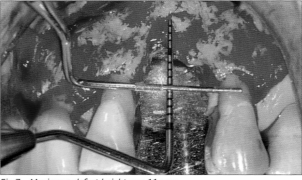

Fig 6   Surgical exposure of the defect.

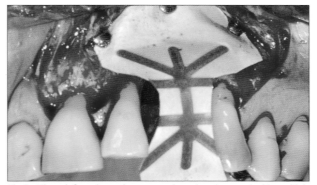

Fig 7   Maximum defect height was 11 mm.

Bone augmentation

Surgery was performed under local anesthesia. Access to the left mandibular ramus was established via an intra-sulcular incision at the second molar and a distal releas-ing incision over the mandibular ramus. This incision is very similar to the approach for thirdmolar surgery, except that the distal incision is more extended. After flap elevation, an adequate quantity of autologous bone chips was harvested with a bone scraper. The flap was then repositioned over the donor site using single silk 5-0 sutures.

A midcrestal incision was performed at the site of the missing canine, including intrasulcular and releasing in-cisions at the adjacent teeth to gain optimal access to the bone defect (Fig 5). After debridement, the true di-mensions of the defect could be appreciated. The buccal and palatal walls were lost, and the maximum vertical dimension of the defect was 11 mm (Figs 6 and 7). Root planing was performed on both the lateral incisor and the premolar.

A Gore-Tex® Titanium Reinforced (Gore® TR9) mem-brane was shaped and adapted to the defect, using ti-tanium pins (FRIOS® membrane tacks, Dentsply) for temporary fixation of the membrane to the buccal bone wall (Fig 8) and a titanium screw (Straumann® Modus, diameter 1.5 mm, length 14 mm) to provide additional stabilization of the membrane in the coronal defect area (Fig 9).

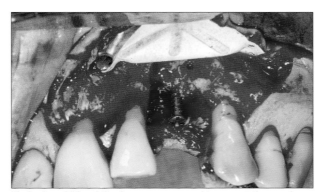

Fig 8   The reinforced membrane was shaped and secured with multiple titanium pins.

Fig 9   An additional titanium screw was used to support the membrane in the central area.

After filling the defect with autologous bone chips, the membrane was closed and secured with supplementary titanium pins. On the palatal side, the membrane was simply stabilized by the palatal flap (Figs 10 to 13). Care was taken to respect a minimum distance of 1.5 mm from the adjacent teeth to reduce the risk of membrane exposure and contamination.

A double layer of a collagen membrane (Bio-Gide®; Geistlich Biomaterials, Wolhusen, Switzerland) was placed on top of the Gore membrane. This technique is supposed to reduce the risks involved in initial soft-tissue healing, notably in the event of wound dehiscence (Fig 14).

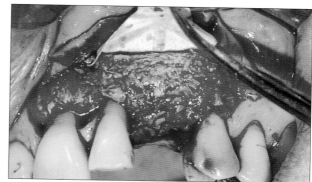

Fig 10   Defect filled with autologous bone chips to restore an ideal ridge shape (labial view).

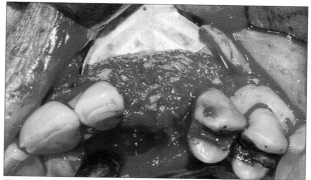

Fig 11   Defect filled with autologous bone chips to restore an ideal ridge shape (occlusal view).

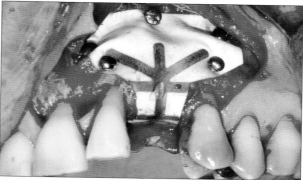

Fig 12   Membrane secured with additional titanium pins (labial view).

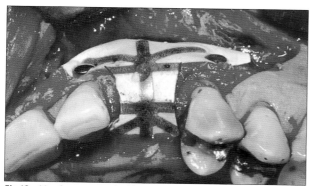

Fig 13   Membrane secured with additional titanium pins (occlusal view).

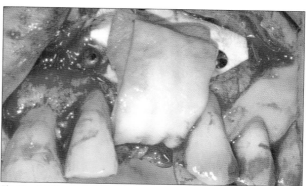

Fig 14   A collagen membrane is placed on the ePTFE membrane.

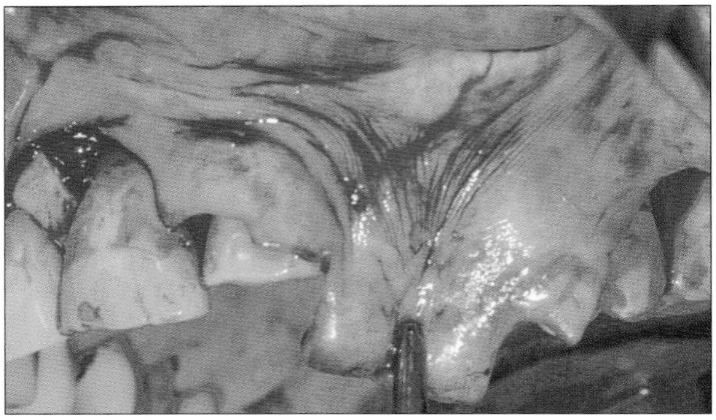

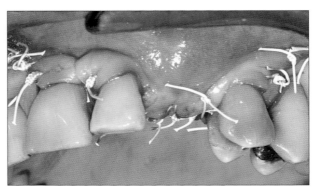

Fig 15   Mobilization of the flap before suturing.

Fig 16   Passive suturing.

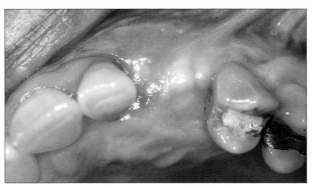

Fig 17   Healing status after 9 months, immediately before implant surgery was begun.

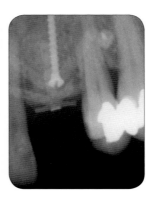

Fig 18 Radiograph demonstrating that the density of the grafted area was adequate.

By interrupting its periosteal layer, the flap could be mobilized and adapted without tension (Fig 15). The flap of the recipient site was finally sutured with single and mattress Gore® 5-0 sutures (Fig 16).

Intake of antibiotics was started on the day before surgery and was continued for 6 days postoperatively. Non-steroidal anti-inflammatory medication and chlorhexidine mouthrinses were prescribed for 3 weeks. The patient was instructed to avoid any kind of mechanical stress in the surgically treated areas.

When the sutures were removed after 15 days, the patient reported no significant symptoms other than swelling.

The temporary bonded restoration was applied after suture removal, avoiding any contact with the surgically treated area.

Implant surgery

Implant surgery was scheduled to take place after 9 months of uneventful healing (Fig 17). The same surgical access was to be used. A preoperative radiograph was obtained, which confirmed good density of the regenerated bone (Fig 18).

After removing the membrane and the Modus screw, an adequate volume of regenerated bone could be verified (Figs 19 to 21). The implant bed was prepared following the usual protocol and a bone-level implant (Bone Level SLActive®, diameter 4.1 mm, length 12 mm; Straumann, Basel, Switzerland) inserted, which was found to be surrounded by an adequate bone volume (Figs 22 and 23).

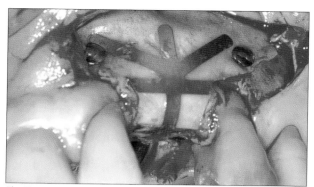

Fig 19 Favorable appearance of the membrane and preservation of the regenerated bone volume.

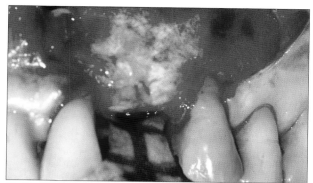

Fig 20 Adequate bone volume (labial view).

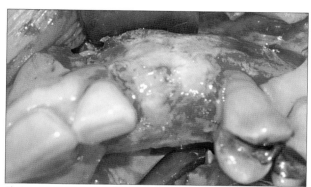

Fig 21 Adequate bone volume (occlusal view).

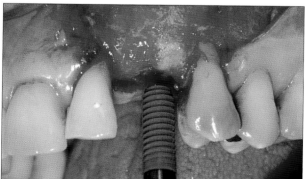

Fig 22 Placement of the implant.

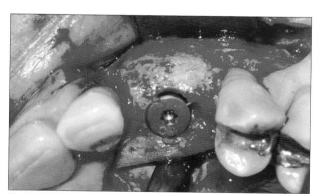

Fig 23 The implant was surrounded by an adequate bone volume.

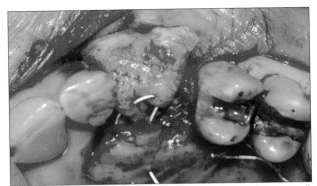

Fig 24   A connective-tissue graft was placed to optimize soft-tissue conditions.

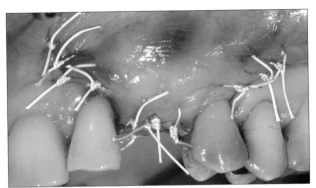

Fig 25   Sutures in place.

This implant design—with its highly osteoconductive and rapidly osseointegrating SLActive® surface—was selected to speed up osseointegration, which is a relevant consideration for time-consuming rehabilitations that involve multiple treatment steps. Bone density was considered adequate, and the implant showed good primary stability.

Soft-tissue management was optimized by augmenting the thickness of the mucosa with a connective-tissue graft placed over the implant site (Fig 24). Primary wound closure was achieved with single ePTFE 5-0 sutures (Fig 25).

Re-entry

Another 2 months of healing were allowed before the re-entry procedure was conducted. This was accomplished by raising a small flap not involving the adjacent papillae and adapting it circumferentially to the healing abutment with thin resorbable 6-0 sutures (Vycril™; Ethicon, Johnson & Johnson Medical, New Brunswick, NJ, USA) (Figs 26 and 27).

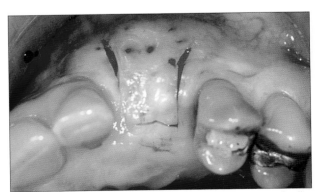

Fig 26   A small flap was used to reopen the site and connect a healing abutment.

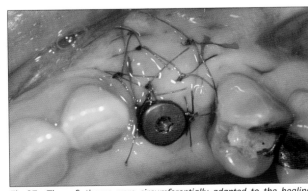

Fig 27   The soft tissues were circumferentially adapted to the healing abutment with 6-0 sutures.

Prosthetic procedures

The phase of prosthetic rehabilitation was initiated 1 week after suture removal by inserting a temporary screw-retained crown whose purpose was to condition the soft tissues.

After 3 months, a new impression was taken and the definitive zirconia crown fabricated. This implant-supported crown was cemented onto a Straumann titanium abutment tightened to the implant to a torque of 35 Ncm. A non-eugenol, acrylic-urethane, polymer-based cement for implant luting (Implacem®; Dentalica, Milan, Italy) was used (Fig 28). A definitive glass-ionomer cement was used to deliver the crown for the residual tooth structure at the adjacent site 24. A final periapical radiograph was obtained, which confirmed that the final restorations were correctly adapted (Fig 29).

The definitive appearance of the treated area and its esthetics in the patient's smile may be considered highly acceptable compared to the initial situation (Figs 30 and 31). As had been anticipated, the preexisting bone loss at the teeth adjacent to the missing canine had prevented complete elimination of the little black triangles in the interproximal spaces.

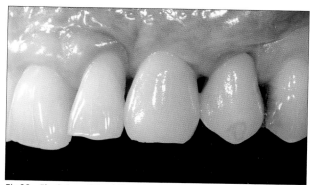

Fig 28   Final view of the delivered crowns.

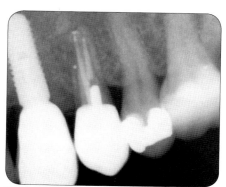

Fig 29   Final radiograph for verification.

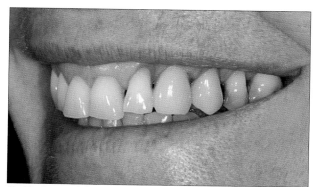

Fig 30   Extraoral view of the patient's improved smile.

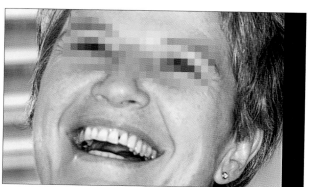

Fig 31   Portrait view of the patient's smile.

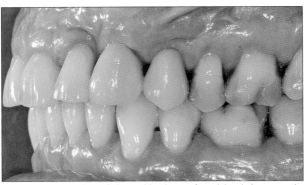

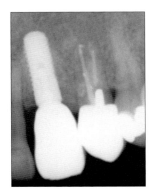

Fig 33   Radiograph at the 1-year follow-up.

Fig 32   Good stability of the peri-implant soft and hard tissues at the 1-year follow-up.

Periodic follow-up and professional maintenance visits were scheduled at 6-month intervals with radiographs to be obtained every year.

The follow-up visit after 1 year revealed no signs of inflammation in the peri-implant soft tissues and no significant bone resorption associated with the implant (Figs 32 and 33). The patient was perfectly satisfied with the esthetics and function of her rehabilitation.

Acknowledgments

Prosthetic procedures
Dr. Martin Tschurtschenthaler – Bruneck, Italy

Laboratory procedures
Anton Maierunteregger – Bruneck, Italy

6.4 Autologous Block Graft and Guided Bone Regeneration (GBR) for Horizontal Ridge Augmentation in the Posterior Mandible

D. Buser, B. Schmid

An 18-year-old man was referred for implant therapy in the posterior mandible to the Department of Oral Surgery and Stomatology (University of Bern, Switzerland). He was healthy and did not smoke. Tooth 35 was congenitally missing, involving a single-tooth edentulous space that offered an adequate mesiodistal dimension for implant placement but exhibited a typical pattern of buccal flattening. A panoramic radiograph was obtained, which revealed a sufficient vertical bone height above the mandibular canal and a normal bone structure in the edentulous area (Fig 1).

After discussing the situation with the patient, it was agreed to proceed with the following treatment plan:

- Horizontal ridge augmentation of site 35 with an autologous block and GBR
- Five months later, implant placement into the augmented ridge
- Restoration with an implant-supported single crown

Following elevation of a mucoperiosteal flap, the local anatomy exhibited a crest narrower than 3 mm. This meant that an implant could not be inserted to its correct position simultaneously with GBR (Fig 2).

Instead, it was decided to augment the horizontal ridge dimension with a block graft harvested from the chin area. This corticocancellous graft was applied to the buccal bone surface and stabilized with a self-tapping miniscrew (Fig 3) to achieve a new crest width of roughly 8 mm.

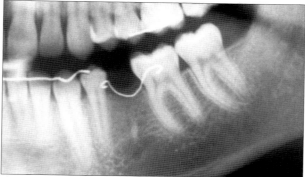

Fig 1   Panoramic radiograph of the single-tooth gap in the posterior mandible. Both the mesiodistal space and the bone height above the mental foramen were sufficient to place an implant.

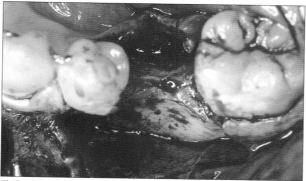

Fig 2   Buccal flattening was clearly apparent under the elevated flap. The crest was less than 3 mm wide, too narrow to place an implant in its correct position.

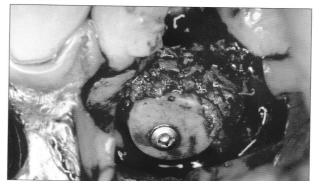

Fig 3   The block graft used for horizontal augmentation was stabilized with a screw. A mixture of DBBM particles and bone chips was used to fill the voids around the block graft.

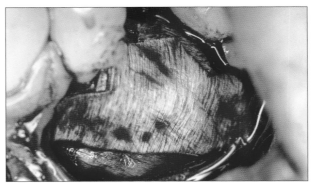

Fig 4   The augmentation material was covered with a collagen membrane to create a temporary barrier for the duration of wound healing.

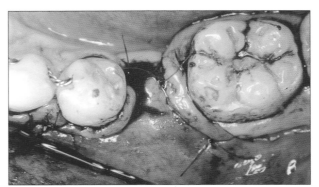

Fig 5   Surgery was finalized by tension-free primary wound closure. Note that a midcrestal incision could be used to facilitate the surgical procedure.

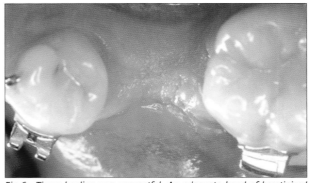

Fig 6   Tissue healing was uneventful. An adequate band of keratinized mucosa was available at the future implant site 35, requiring a slightly lingual incision line for the second surgery.

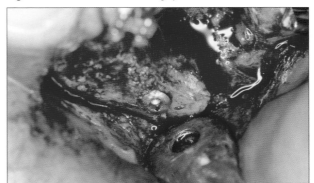

Fig 7   Buccal view during the second surgery. The block graft was well integrated and showed no signs of resorption.

Small bone chips, which had been locally harvested, were mixed with deproteinized bovine bone mineral (DBBM) available in particulated form as Bio-Oss® (Geistlich Biomaterials, Wolhusen, Switzerland) to fill the voids surrounding the block graft (Fig 4). In keeping with the concept of GBR, the augmentation material was then covered with a resorbable collagen membrane (Bio-Gide®; Geistlich Biomaterials).

Tension-free primary wound closure was established to complete the first surgery. It is important to note that it was possible to use a midcrestal incision for this surgical procedure (Fig 5). Postsurgical healing was uneventful (Fig 6).

The second procedure was performed after 5 months of healing. Following flap elevation, the block graft was found to be well integrated and—as indicated by the position of the miniscrew head—exhibited no signs of surface resorption (Fig 7).

Given the new crest width of about 8 mm, a wide-diameter implant with a diameter of 4.8 mm could be selected. The implant bed was prepared and found to have a facial bone wall roughly 2 mm in thickness (Fig 8). Good primary stability was achieved upon inserting the selected 10-mm tissue-level implant (Straumann, Basel, Switzerland).

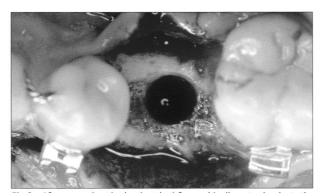

Fig 8   After preparing the implant bed for a wide-diameter implant, the resultant thickness of the buccal bone wall was around 2 mm.

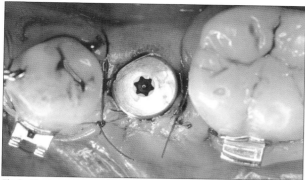

Fig 9   Surgery was completed by closing the wound for non-submerged healing.

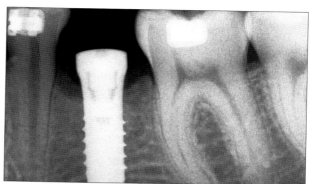

Fig 10   Postsurgical radiograph. Correct position and proper angulation of the wide-diameter implant.

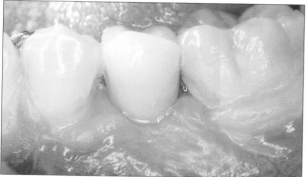

Fig 11   After 8 weeks of healing, the well-integrated implant was restored with a cemented crown.

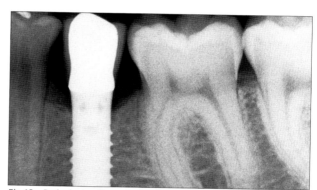

Fig 12   Periapical radiograph. Excellent integration of the implant and a good fit between the implant and the crown.

After fitting the implant with a 2-mm healing cap, the wound margins were adapted for non-submerged healing. Two interrupted single sutures were used to secure the soft tissues (Fig 9). A postsurgical radiograph was obtained to verify the position and angulation of the 10-mm implant (Fig 10).

Following 8 weeks of uneventful healing, a single crown was cemented onto the implant (Figs 11 and 12).

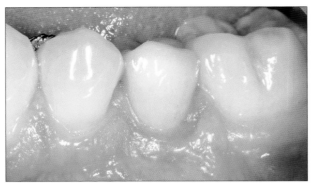

Fig 13   Clinical view at the 10-year follow-up. Healthy peri-implant mu-cosa and nice band of keratinized tissue.

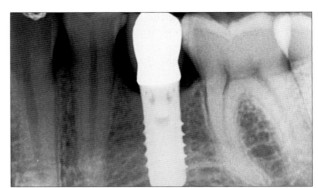

Fig 14   Radiograph at the 10-year follow up. Excellent stability of the cr-estal bone levels mesial and distal to the implant.

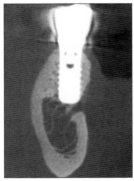

Fig 15   Orofacial CBCT view at the 10-year follow-up. The implant was well integrated and associated with a fully intact buccal bone wall.

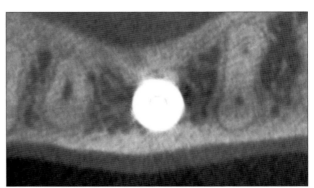

Fig 16   Horizontal CBCT view at the 10-year follow-up. Successful long-term outcome of horizontal ridge augmentation.

The patient was scheduled for an aftercare maintenance program. At the 10-year follow-up visit, the clinical status was characterized by healthy and keratinized mucosa (Fig 13). A periapical radiograph revealed stable levels of the peri-implant crestal bone (Fig 14), and an additional CBCT scan (4 × 4 cm) confirmed the presence of an intact facial bone wall (around 1.5 mm thick) at the implant site (Figs 15 and 16).

Discussion

Treatment of this patient included a resorbable collagen membrane to cover a block graft that had been applied for horizontal ridge augmentation. Our group started using this type of membrane around 2000—after a preclinical study had yielded promising results (Hürzeler and coworkers 1998)—to replace the biologically inert non-resorbable membranes of the expanded polytetrafluoroethylene (ePTFE) type (Gore-Tex® Regenerative Membrane; W.L. Gore & Associates, Flagstaff, AZ, USA).

While ePTFE membranes did offer good regenerative outcomes of horizontal ridge augmentation (Buser and coworkers 1996), their use was associated with a highly demanding surgical technique (notably in the mandible). Among other drawbacks, they required a beveled two-layer incision on the buccal side to avoid postoperative soft-tissue dehiscence (Buser and coworkers 1995).

The possibility of using a midcrestal incision technique with the introduction of collagen membranes clearly simplified the surgical approach. A prospective case series of 42 patients demonstrated that collagen membranes yielded the same good results as ePTFE membranes placed over block grafts while greatly reducing the difficults level of the surgical technique (von Arx and Buser 2006; von Arx and Buser 2009).

Today there would also be option of considering a narrow-diameter implant made of a titanium-zirconia alloy (Roxolid®; Straumann, Basel, Switzerland) in clinical situations such as the one presented here. This novel material reduces the risk of implant fracture by offering increased strength (Kobayashi and coworkers 1995). Narrow-diameter implants are an interesting option especially for premolar sites in the mandible, which commonly present with borderline anatomical conditions (Braut and coworkers 2012). Also, they can often pave the way for a simplified surgical protocol by allowing GBR to be conducted simultaneously with implant placement (Buser 2009). Short-term experience with narrow-diameter implants made of Roxolid® have yielded promising results (Al-Nawas and coworkers 2012; Barter and coworkers 2012; Chiapasco and coworkers 2012). Therefore, while caution should still be exercised, their use may be considered in clinical situations of this type.

6.5   Autologous Iliac-Crest Graft for Anterior Blocks and Bilateral Sinus Floor Elevation in a Completely Edentulous Maxilla

W. D. Polido, P. E. Pittas do Canto

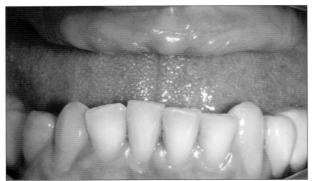

Fig 1   Initial clinical presentation of the edentulous maxilla.

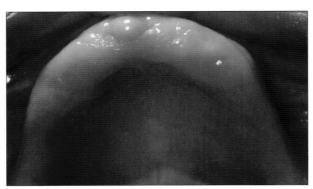

Fig 2   Initial clinical presentation (occlusal view).

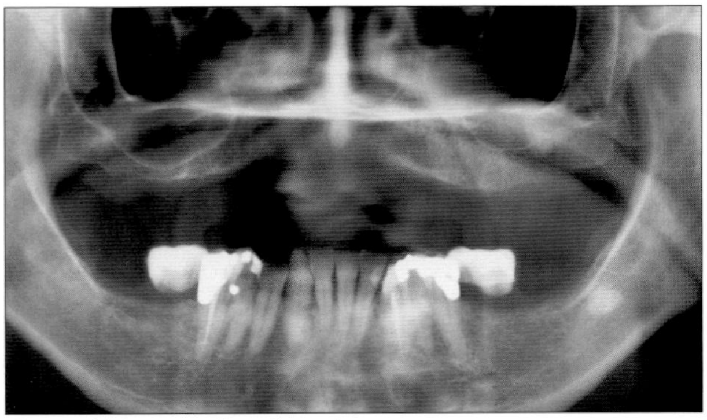

A 56-year-old woman presented for treatment with complete edentulism of the maxilla. She had been using a complete removable denture since she was relatively young (age 30). Her chief complaint at presentation was lack of retention of the upper denture and a desire for a better restoration in order to improve retention, function, and esthetics.

An initial clinical examination showed that the anterior maxilla was moderately atrophic both horizontally and vertically, also revealing a vertical deficiency of the posterior alveolar process (Figs 1 and 2). The mandible included natural teeth from 45 to 35, with previous extrusion of the anterior teeth that was being orthodontically treated. Also, there were two external hexagon dental implants at sites 46 and 36 that had been inserted elsewhere at a previous point in time. As the conditions in the mandible were healthy, including the teeth and the two implants, the patient had no complaints there.

The patient provided a panoramic radiograph that showed her condition before orthodontic treatment and placement of the mandibular implants (Fig 3).

![Initial panoramic radiograph]

Fig 3   Initial panoramic radiograph.

Computed tomography showed a lack of bone thickness in the anterior maxilla and lack of height in the posterior maxilla (Figs 4a-d).

Treatment options

Three different treatment options were presented to the patient:

- Placement of four implants, including two narrower but longer tissue-level implants (Soft Tissue Level RN, diameter 3.3 mm, length 10 mm; Straumann, Basel, Switzerland) in the anterior maxilla with possible simultaneous guided bone regeneration, and two wider but shorter tissue-level implants (Soft Tissue Level RN, diameter 4.1 mm, length 8 mm; Straumann) in the posterior maxilla with osteotome techniques for sinus floor elevation. Restoration would feature a removable overdenture; however, the posterior height on the right side was very limited for the osteotome technique, and a sinus floor elevation or tilted implants would have to be used.
- Grafting of the anterior maxilla with a mandibular ramus block and of the posterior maxilla with a mixture of autologous bone chips and bone substitute. After six months of healing, six implants would potentially be placed in order to restore the maxilla with a complete fixed prosthesis featuring pink restorative material to compensate for the lack of alveolar bone and to add esthetics and lip support. The idea of combining bone substitute and autologous ramus grafts was very novel at the time (2004). Also, the use of a complete maxillary prosthesis with a large pink component would make dental hygiene more difficult (especially in aging patients), and fixed complete prostheses with splinting of all implants are more prone to cause maintenance problems than segmented bridges.
- Placement of an iliac crest bone graft in a completely edentulous maxilla using anterior corticocancellous blocks and bilateral sinus floor elevation with a lateral window technique, to obtain an ideal three-dimensional reconstruction of the alveolar atrophy. Grafting would be followed by placement of eight implants to deliver four three-unit fixed partial dentures 4 to 5 months later.

After discussing all the risks and benefits of the treatment choices, the patient's decision was in favor of the iliac-crest reconstruction. Key factors motivating her to opt for the procedure that had held the highest promise in terms of outcome included her good general health, young age, and desire for the best possible restorations (also reflected by her willingness to undergo orthodontic treatment in the mandible).

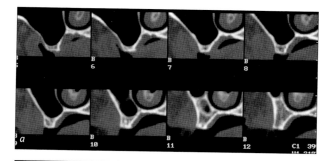
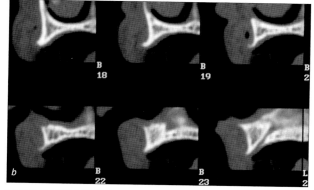
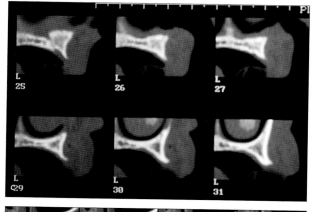
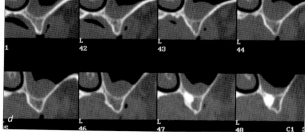

Figs 4a-d   Initial CT scan of the edentulous maxilla.

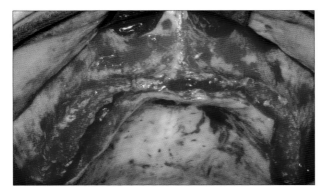

Fig 5   Surgical view of the completely edentulous maxilla.

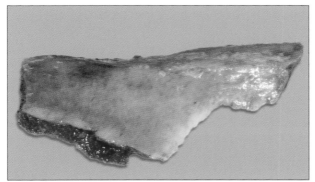

Fig 6   Block graft harvested from the iliac crest.

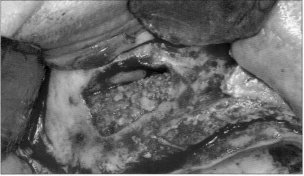

Fig 7   Sinus floor elevation showing a lateral window with bone graft on the right side.

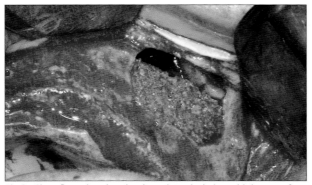

Fig 8   Sinus floor elevation showing a lateral window with bone graft on the left side. Notice the cortical perforations in the anterior maxilla.

Bone harvesting and graft placement

After a complete medical check-up, surgery was performed under general anesthesia in November 2004. Iliac crest bone was harvested from the left hip by the team's orthopedic surgeon simultaneously with maxillofacial surgery. Care was taken to harvest bone in a corticocancellous block from the medial aspect, preserving the top of the crest.

In the maxilla, a mucoperiosteal incision was performed on the top of the crest, going from the tuberosity on the right side to the tuberosity region on the left side. Small releasing incisions were made bilaterally on the posterior aspects. Today our preference is to keep the posterior region intact and to make a releasing incision in the midline (Kleinheinz and coworkers 2005).

After complete and careful subperiosteal reflection of the flap, exposure of the anterior wall of the maxilla was achieved. Reflection was carried upward until complete exposure of the infraorbital foramen, and posteriorly to the tuberosities. This wide subperiosteal reflection facilitates later mobilization of the flap, minimizing the need for periosteal releasing incisions, maintaining vascularization to the graft, as well as achieving passive closure of the wound (Fig 5).

Next, a round diamond drill was used for sinus floor elevation with the lateral window technique, as described by Katsuyama and Jensen (2011) (Figs 7 and 8). All traditional steps of sinus floor elevation were followed through on both sides of the maxilla. There were no complications.

At the same time, one member of our maxillofacial team was already preparing the bone blocks harvested by the orthopedic surgeon.

As soon as we had the rough blocks (Fig 6), measurements were taken with calipers in the anterior maxilla to achieve the best adaptation of the graft. The blocks were carefully sculpted with continuous checking of size and position. Care was taken not to compress the nasal mucosa.

A remaining part of the corticocancellous block, as well as part of the cancellous bone curetted from the hip, was milled with a R. Quétin Bone Mill device (R. Quétin Dental Products, Leimen, Germany) to be used for packing in the sinus-floor elevation graft and around the blocks after fixation.

Using a flexible thin and large spatula to protect the elevated sinus mucosa and to prevent loose chips of bone from getting into the sinus, bone was condensed toward the anterior and inferior region. Complete condensation is important, as this will result in less resorption and a better quality of bone regeneration. A larger quantity of cancellous bone is preferred.

After packing of the sinus graft on the right side, corticocancellous blocks were positioned and stabilized with bicortical screws 1.6 × 10 and 1.6 × 12 mm (Osteomed Mincro, Addison, TX, USA) (Fig 9), starting from the anterior segment and moving to the right posterior segment, and then to the left posterior segment.

Prior to positioning the anterior corticocancellous grafts, small perforations with a round bur (size ¼) were created in the cortical wall of the anterior maxilla for decorticalization and improved vascularization of the host bed. Then a portion of cancellous graft was packed into the host area. As soon as the blocks were positioned with the cortical part facing the buccal and occlusal aspects, the grafts were fixated using the lag-screw (compressive) technique, squeezing the cancellous bone against the walls to eliminate any gaps between the block graft and the host site. Before securing the grafts, minor compression of the cancellous area was achieved to eliminate some of the fat content and reduce the lacunae. We consider these two steps very important and among the key prerequisites for successful grafting (excellent integration and less resorption).

With the grafts held in place with a clamp, two 1.6 × 12 mm fixation screws (Osteomed Mincro, Addison TX, USA) were positioned in each block, again using the lag-screw compressive technique. The 1.0-mm drill was used to perforate the graft and recipient site and the 1.3-mm drill to perforate just the graft. It is important that the screw is long enough to engage the host site without perforating the palatal mucosa. After perforation, the screw size can be measured with a depth gauge.

Care was taken to adapt the block completely without leaving any gaps. The distal fixation screw was placed through the anterior wall of the sinus. When it was completed and the block was stable, the anterior block on the opposite side was positioned.

Once all blocks were fixated, any prominent edges of the bone were rounded off with a round or piriform trimming bur, and remaining cancellous bone was packed around the blocks to fill any existing gaps (Figs 10 to 12).

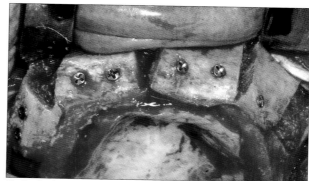
Fig 9   Corticocancellous blocks were adapted to the anterior maxilla and stabilized with screws.

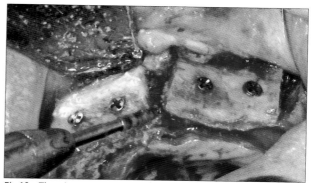
Fig 10   The edges were rounded with a pear-shaped bur.

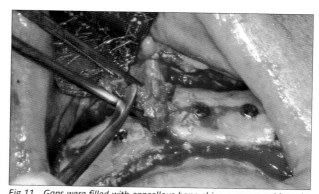
Fig 11   Gaps were filled with cancellous bone chips, compressed into the remaining spaces.

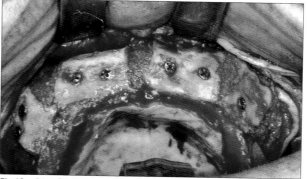
Fig 12   Gaps filled completely with autologous bone chips.

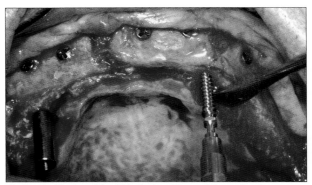

Fig 13   Positioning of the IPI in the basal bone of the canine site.

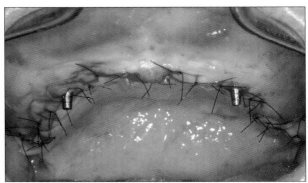

Fig 14   Complete closure of the wound. Notice the posts of the IPIs.

Placement of provisional implants

After all blocks were stable, we placed two one-piece machined-surface provisional implants (Immediate Provisional Implants, IPI; diameter 2.8 mm, length 13.6 mm; Nobel Biocare, Göteborg, Sweden) in the remaining alveolar bone of the canine region (Figs 13 and 14). Their purpose was to assist in supporting the denture after surgery without compressing the graft. It is important to place these provisional implants on the patient's own remaining alveolar process, which is now more palatally oriented, and not on the graft itself. There is an increased risk of graft contamination through the IPI, leading to increased resorption around the IPI area, loss of bone, and loss of the provisional implant (Castagna and coworkers 2013).

Careful soft-tissue closure is of utmost importance. We performed subperiosteal dissection as apically as possible, going laterally to the piriform aperture and almost as high as the infraorbital foramen. By dissecting subperiosteally rather than incising, we can get a good soft-tissue release and maintain periosteal integrity. If necessary, small periosteal incisions are performed first internally in the periosteum along the releasing incisions done distally, without cutting through the mucosa). Complete and passive soft-tissue adaptation without ex-

cessive pull or incisions is important. We considered this another critical surgical step.

Closing of the flap was performed with 4-0 mononylon sutures, which were removed 15 days after the surgery. The patient agreed to postpone wearing the removable partial denture to avoid soft-tissue compression for 7 days.

Pre- and postoperative medication

As part of our routine protocol for iliac-crest grafts, patients receive intravenous medication during their 48-hour hospital stay. This includes antibiotics (cefazolin 1 g i.v. every 8 hours) and anti-inflammatory drugs (dexamethasone 10 mg i.v. every 12 hours and tramadol i.v. every 6 hours). After hospital discharge, patients continue with cefadroxil 500 mg every 12 hours for 7 days, a non-steroidal ant-inflammatory drug every 8 hours for 5 days and, if necessary, a strong analgesic. Chlorhexidine oral rinses are prescribed for 3 weeks.

Provisionalization and graft healing

After 7 to 10 days, the removable denture was adjusted to reduce its volume, and a soft relining material was added. A recommendation was given to the patient to reduce the time of wearing the denture as much as possible and to sleep without it.

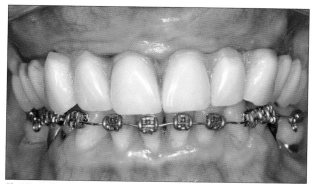

Fig 15   Follow-up view 4 months after surgery, showing adaptation of the provisional denture. Notice the complete absence of the anterior flange.

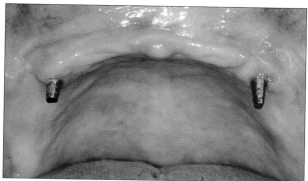

Fig 16   Occlusal view of the maxilla 4 months after grafting. There was nice soft-tissue healing around the IPIs.

The sutures were removed around 20 days after surgery, once complete soft-tissue healing was noted. The soft reliner material was reapplied and trimmed to avoid pressure over the graft. The occlusion was adjusted to avoid excessive compression (Figs 15 and 16).

One month after the graft surgery, the patient started to take sodium alendronate 70 mg perorally once a week until the implants would be loaded (usually 4 to 6 months after grafting). This medication approach reduces bone resorption and increases bone density, improving the quality of the bone for implant placement. The use of alendronate is discontinued once the restorations have been placed and the implants loaded.

Recently it has been discussed in the literature (Oates 2013) that short-term use of low-potency bisphosphonates may prove to be useful in reducing graft resorption and improving bone density without the risks of jaw osteonecrosis associated with intravenous application of bisphosphonates at higher doses and over longer periods. Having used this approach without any complications since 2002, we have found it to yield excellent results in terms of long-term resorption control and graft volume preservation.

Revisions are made once a month, with re-adaptation of the denture and inspection of soft-tissue healing. If required, denture adhesives (strips or paste) may be used to improve denture stability during the healing phase.

Five months after the grafting procedure, with uneventful healing, a new CT image was taken (Figs 17 and 18a-e), showing a complete adaptation of the graft and the volume of the three-dimensional reconstruction. Soft-tissue adaptation was also considered very good.

Leveling of the lower arch by orthodontic treatment was also achieved.

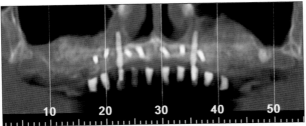

Fig 17   *CT scan of the maxilla 5 months after grafting. A simple radiographic guide was used, with a radiopaque material (in this case gutta-percha) placed in the palatal aspect of each tooth in the provisional denture.*

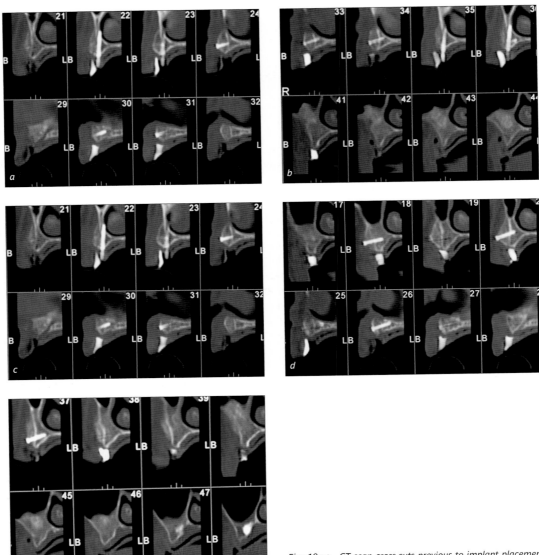

Figs 18a-e   *CT scan cross-cuts previous to implant placement surgery.*

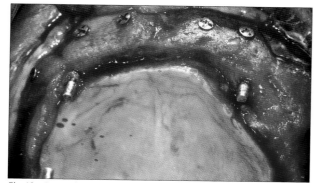

Fig 19 Bone view at implant placement. Remodeling, but only minor resorption.

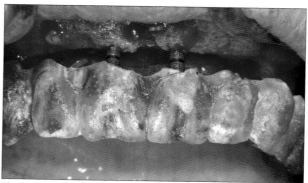

Fig 20 Intraoperative view of the surgical guide and its relationship to the facial midline and direction indicator pins.

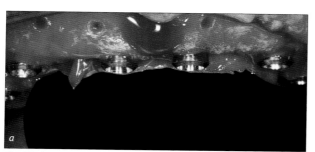

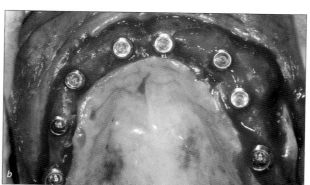

Figs 21a-b Occlusal and anterior view of the implant positions during surgery.

Restoration with implants

Implant and restorative choices were again discussed with the patient. Six implants and a complete twelve-unit prosthesis were the first choice, but eight implants and four three-unit fixed partial dentures was a good option after the success of the grafts. The advantages of this restorative choice have been discussed in Volume 4 of the ITI Treatment Guide (Casentini and coworkers 2010; Gallucci and coworkers 2010).

After diagnostic waxing and construction of a surgical splint, the decision was made to place eight implants in regions 16, 14, 13, 11, 21, 23, 24, and 26, under local anesthesia:

- 16, 26 – Tapered Effect WN, SLA, diameter 4.8 mm, length 10 mm
- 14, 24 – Tapered Effect RN, SLA, diameter 4.1 mm, length 10 mm
- 13, 23 – Tapered Effect RN, SLA, diameter 4.1 mm, length 12 mm
- 11, 21 – Tapered Effect RN, SLA, diameter 4.1 mm, length 10 mm

At the time of treatment, only the soft-tissue level SLA implants were available. Today we would consider

the use of Bone Level SLActive® implants in this kind of situation. Smaller-diameter implants with the platform-switch connection may be beneficial for preserving alveolar bone in these reconstruction cases. A Bone Level Regular CrossFit® for the posterior areas and a Bone Level Narrow CrossFit® for the anterior areas would be the indication for a similar case today. (All implants Straumann, Basel, Switzerland.)

Implant surgery was performed under local anesthesia in March 2005, with removal of the fixation screws and placement of the implants. Thanks to the previously used surgical technique, little remodeling and resorption had taken place by the time of implant surgery (Fig 19).

When doing implant surgery in these cases, it is important to position the central incisors in precise relation to the patient's midline, as discussed by Ellis and Mc-Fadden (2007). A surgical guide is very important, but securing and positioning it in the correct place is not always easy and may lead to a false impression of correct positioning (Fig 20).

Bone density was excellent, allowing for a single-stage technique and a 6- to 8-week osseointegration period, which is normal with the SLActive® surface (Fig 21).

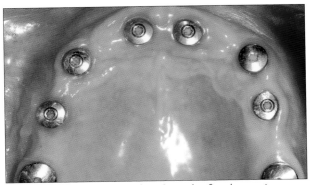

Fig 22   Occlusal view of the implants 3 months after placement.

Postsurgical follow-up

After 8 weeks, impressions were taken. The restorative procedures, including provisionals, took around 6 months to be completed due to the patient's personal commitments (Figs 22 and 23a-b).

In January 2006, four three-unit, cement-retained, metal-ceramic, fixed partial dentures were placed using solid abutments. On the radiographs, a small gap could be noticed on implants 13 and 23 (Figs 24 to 27a-b).

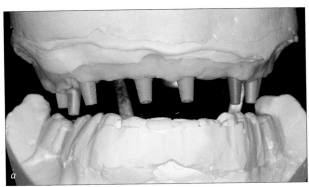
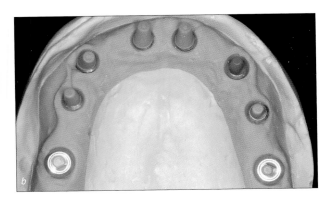

Figs 23a-b   Abutment selection, models.

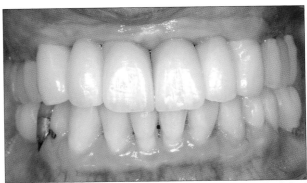

Fig 24   Final restorations included four three-unit, cement-retained, fixed partial dentures. Frontal view in occlusion.

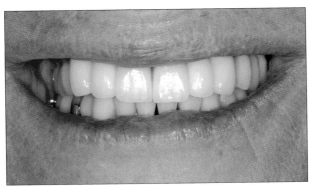

Fig 25   Smile line.

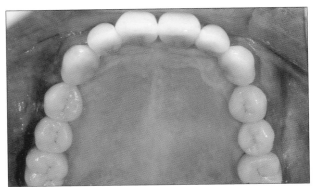

Fig 26   Occlusal view.

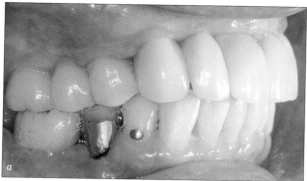
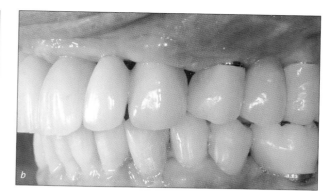

Figs 27a-b   Occlusion on the right (a) and left (b).

The patient came in for follow-up 6 months later, and although the periapical radiograph still showed a small gap, the clinical aspect was very good, with no signs of inflammation.

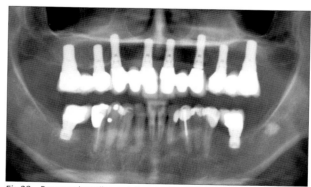

Fig 28   Panoramic radiograph 1 year after restoration.

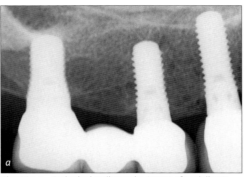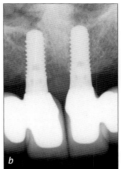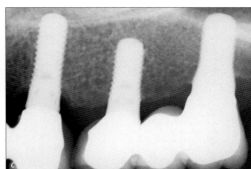

Figs 29a-c Periapical radiographs 1 year after delivery.

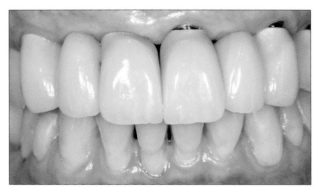

Fig 30 Clinical view at the 6-year follow-up, showing occlusion.

The patient was temporarily lost to follow-up for several reasons, but we could get her to return in 2012. The 6-year follow-up is shown, with periapical radiographs and a cone-beam computed tomography (CBCT) scan (Figs 29a-c to 36a-f).

The gap was still present, with no signs of clinical inflammation. There was no bone resorption, and the result was stable after 6 years.

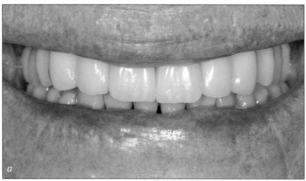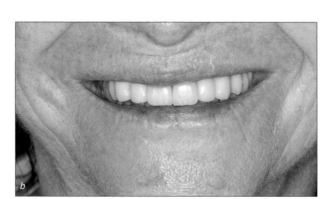

Figs 31a-b Smile line.

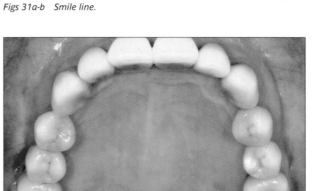

Fig 32 Occlusal view.

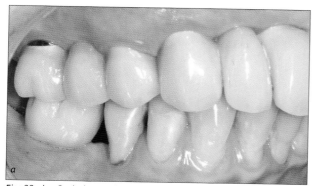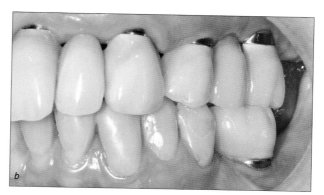

Figs 33a-b   Occlusion on the right (a) and left (b).

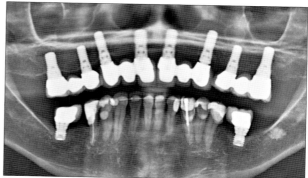

Fig 34   Panoramic radiograph 6 years after delivery.

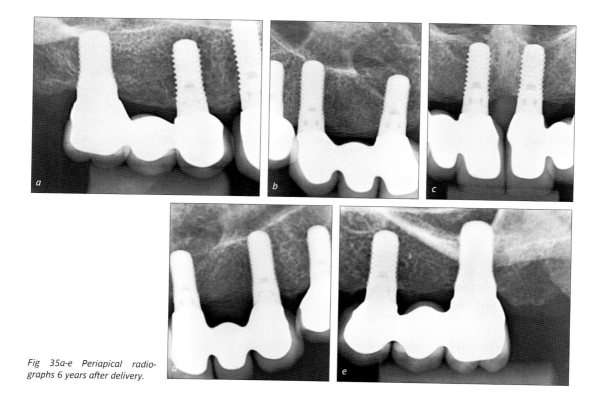

Fig 35a-e   Periapical radiographs 6 years after delivery.

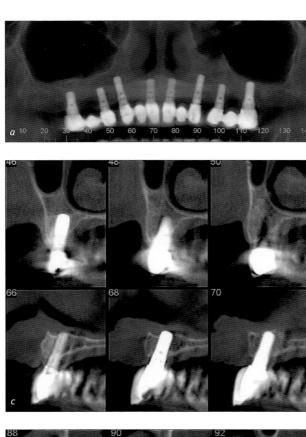

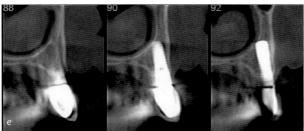

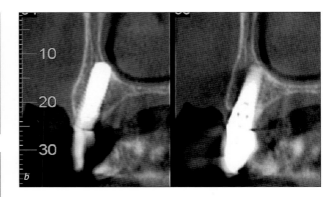

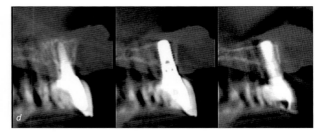

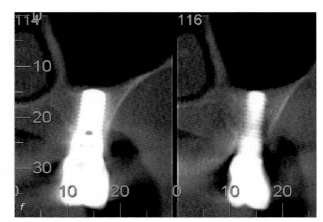

Figs 36a-f   CBCT scan 6 years after delivery.

Acknowledgments

**Orthopedic surgery procedures
(iliac-crest graft harvesting)**
Felipe Wildt do Canto, MD – Porto Alegre, RS, Brazil

Prosthodontic procedures
Paulo Eduardo Pittas do Canto, DDS,
Prosthetic Dentistry – Porto Alegre, RS, Brazil

Dental laboratory procedures
Dental Lab – Porto Alegre, RS, Brazil

The authors also would like to thank Dr. Angelo Menuci Neto, DDS, MS, for his assistance during treatment of the patient, conducted with post-graduate students of the Implant Dentistry program at ABO-RS, coordinated by Dr. Polido during the period that the patient was treated.

6.6 Ridge Preservation and Implant Placement for a Fixed Dental Prosthesis After a Car Accident

M. Roccuzzo

It is well known to clinicians that any removal of teeth will, over time, cause the dimensions of the alveolar ridge to be reduced by resorption of the bundle bone and by changes related to external modeling. This development is particularly evident in the crestal region with its thin buccal bone that consists of bundle bone almost entirely. The facial bone will rapidly resorb as blood supply from the periodontal ligament gets disrupted (Araújo and Lindhe 2005). There is no reason why traumatic tooth loss should not have the same consequences.

It takes more than achieving implant osseointegration for a treatment outcome to be considered successful. No deficiency of bone or soft tissue is acceptable when an ideal esthetic outcome is the goal. Several articles (Sanz and coworkers 2011; Vignoletti and coworkers 2011) have reported on techniques of improving the alveolar ridge for implant treatment, notably focusing on protecting tissues from resorption. These techniques should be remembered particularly in patients, such as the one presented in this case report, who for some reason lost several teeth at a time.

An 18-year-old woman was referred for treatment in December 2006. A few days before, she had suffered a severe car accident and lost her teeth 12, 14, 15, 16, and 17 and sustained a complete crown fracture of tooth 13 in the incident (Figs 1 to 3). The clinical examination revealed a medium to high smile line (associated with gingival display in the upper incisor area), a number of fragments, and inflamed soft tissues.

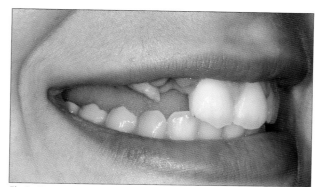

Fig 1   Pretreatment view of the patient's smile.

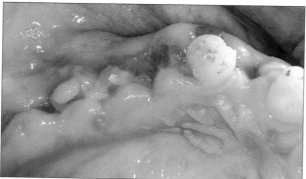

Fig 2   Initial clinical situation around 1 month after the car accident.

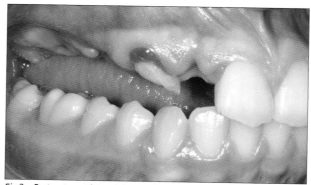

Fig 3   Pretreatment lateral view. Soft-tissue recession in the posterior maxilla and inflammation around the root of the canine.

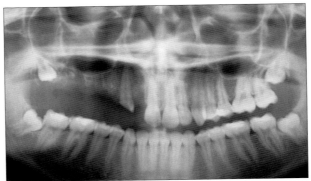

Fig 4   *Panoramic radiograph displaying the canine root, bone atrophy in the posterior maxilla, and residual fragments.*

A panoramic radiograph confirmed that most mandibular right teeth were missing, also revealing an impacted third molar, a fractured canine, and several impacted fragments (Fig 4).

A priority objective was to minimize the risk of excessive horizontal resorption at the esthetically sensitive site 12. An attempt at site preservation in January 2007 included the use of a bovine-derived xenograft (Bio-Oss® collagen, Geistlich Biomaterials, Wolhusen, Switzerland) and a double layer of collagen membrane (Bio-Gide®; Geistlich Biomaterials) for protection. No attempt was made to release the periosteum lest the mucogingival line get coronally displaced. The 4-0 Vicryl™ sutures remained in place for 2 weeks (Figs 5 to 7).

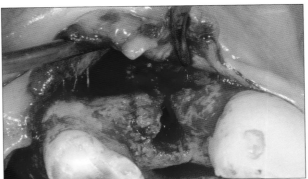

Fig 5   *A small flap was raised to remove residual fragments. Part of the buccal bone plate was missing.*

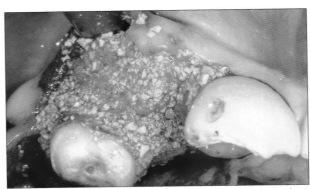

Fig 6   *A composite graft of 10% collagen and deproteinized bovine bone was shaped and inserted into the area.*

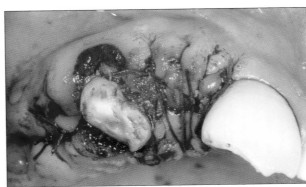

Fig 7   *A double layer of collagen membrane was placed over the grafted area and was secured with Vicryl™ sutures. Care was taken not to displace the mucogingival line coronally.*

A few weeks after placing the xenograft, the patient was referred to a specialist for root canal treatment of the canine. The pertinent radiograph revealed a radiolucent line on the root a few millimeters below the marginal bone crest. The dentist indicated that the tooth could not possibly be preserved but required extraction. Given the patient's compromised general situation, the canine was temporarily kept to facilitate the overall treatment (Figs 8a-b).

The dentist was able to successfully complete the root-canal treatment and to adapt a two-unit fixed provisional restoration after reconstructing the margin of the central incisor (Fig 9).

In May 2007, a traditional procedure of sinus floor elevation (lateral window technique) was conducted to prepare the ground for ideal implant positioning in the posterior maxilla. A staged approach was considered preferable based on the local anatomy and the patient's clinical history (Fig 10). A panoramic radiograph obtained 4 months postoperatively revealed good healing, no radiolucency apical to the canine, and an impacted third molar (Fig 11).

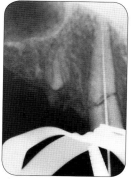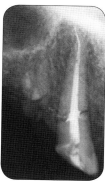

Figs 8a-b   Periapical radiographs obtained during root canal treatment. A root fracture of tooth 13 was noted. It was decided to keep the tooth temporarily for support. (Courtesy of Dr. G. Tessore.)

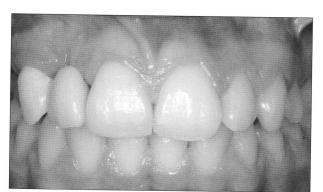

Fig 9   Frontal view after reconstruction of the central incisor and delivery of a two-unit fixed provisional restoration.

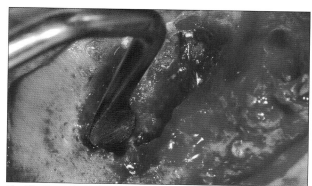

Fig 10   Sinus floor elevation. A lateral window was created and the Schneiderian membrane gently elevated with an appropriate instrument.

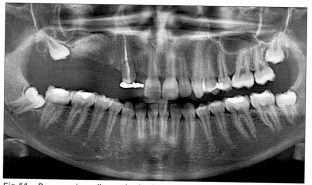

Fig 11   Panoramic radiograph obtained 4 months after sinus floor elevation. Improved vertical dimension distal to the canine.

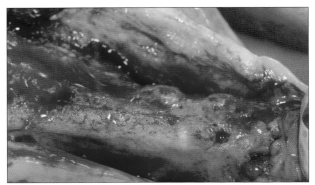

Fig 12   A full-thickness flap was raised distal to the canine.

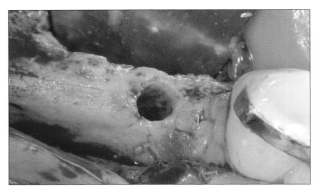

Fig 13   The implant beds were prepared.

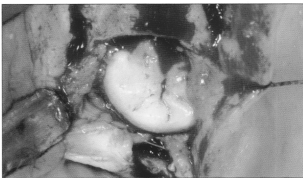

Fig 14   The impacted third molar was removed.

Second-stage surgery for implant placement at sites 14 and 16 (also including extraction of the impacted tooth 18) was performed in November 2007. The procedure took place under local anesthesia and was initiated by performing a midcrestal incision from the distal aspect of the canine to the tuberosity. A full-thickness flap was elevated from the palatal and buccal aspects of the alveolar ridge and was retracted with the aid of sutures (Fig 12). Care was taken to minimize bone loss by employing both drills and osteotomes in preparing the osteotomy sites (Fig 13). The impacted third molar was extracted (Fig 14).

Two titanium implants (Standard Plus RN SLActive®, diameter 4.1 mm, length 10 mm; Straumann, Basel, Switzerland) were placed at the sites of the first premolar and first molar (Fig 15). To reduce the risk of soft- tissue recession notably on the buccal implant surfaces, a bovine-derived xenograft (Bio-Oss® collagen; Geistlich Biomaterials, Wolhusen, Switzerland) was applied to the crest and covered with a collagen membrane (Bio-Gide®; Geistlich Biomaterials) for protection (Figs 16 and 17). Interrupted Vycril™ sutures were used for transmucosal healing. Beveled healing caps were used to facilitate close adaptation of the flap in the interproximal area (Fig 18).

The lateral view obtained 3 months postoperatively demonstrates that horizontal tissue support was excellent (Fig 19).

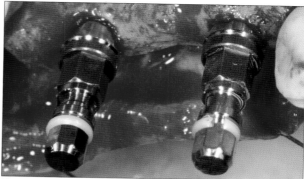

Fig 15 Two Regular Neck implants were placed at the sites of the first premolar and first molar.

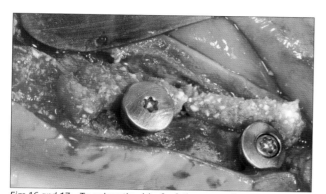

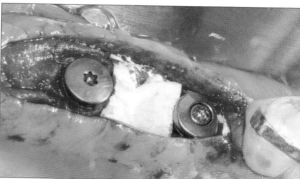

Figs 16 and 17 To reduce the risk of soft-tissue recession around the implants, the grafted area was covered with a double layer of collagen membrane.

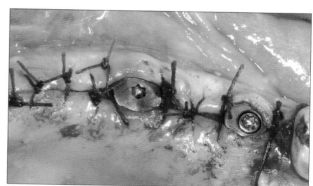

Fig 18 Interrupted Vicryl™ sutures were used for transmucosal healing.

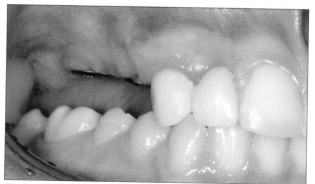

Fig 19 Lateral view obtained 3 months postoperatively. Horizontal tissue support was excellent.

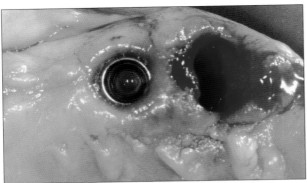

Fig 20   Extraction of the fractured canine and site preservation.

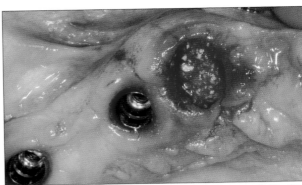

Fig 21   The socket was filled with bovine-derived xenograft (Bio-Oss® collagen).

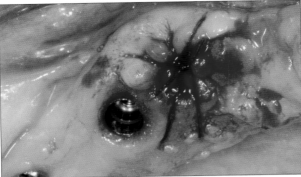

Fig 22   The site was covered with a flowable polylactide polymer and then sutured.

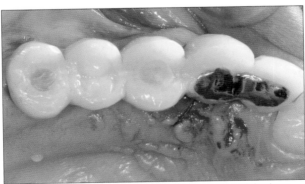

Fig 23   The provisional fixed prosthesis was screwed to both implants.

The canine was extracted once the two implants were capable of predictably supporting a fixed multi-unit provisional prosthesis (Fig 20). To minimize the resultant loss of buccolingual dimension, the socket was filled with bovine-derived xenograft (Bio-Oss® collagen, Geistlich Biomaterials, Wolhusen, Switzerland) (Fig 21). A flowable polylactide polymer (Atrisorb® FreeFlow™; Tolmar Inc., Fort Collins, CO, USA) was used to cover the site and prevent any mobilization of bone substitute particles. Once applied, the barrier was solidified by misting with a fine spray of sterile saline, followed by suturing (Fig 22). Subsequently, a five-unit fixed provisional prosthesis, including two mesial cantilevers, was screwed to the implants at sites 14 and 16 (Fig 23). The patient was finally able to use her first quadrant for chewing and did have acceptable esthetics restored (Fig 24).

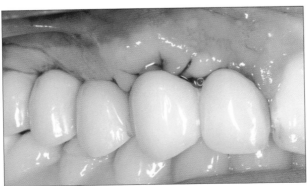

Fig 24   Frontal view of the provisional immediately after surgery.

One more implant was placed at site 12 (Fig 25). This procedure took place 1 year after site preservation, immediately after soft-tissue healing above the canine site. Given the limited amount of bone available at the site, a Narrow Neck implant (Standard Plus NN SLActive®, diameter 3.3 mm, length 10 mm; Straumann, Basel, Switzerland) was selected (Fig 26).

A panoramic radiograph obtained 12 weeks after the procedure confirmed that the implant positions were ideal and that no radiolucencies or other pathologies were present (Fig 27).

The fabrication process for the new five-unit fixed provisional prosthesis, now to be supported by three rather than two implants, was started by taking an impression with the help of screw-on impression caps (Fig 28). Several weeks were allowed for adequate soft-tissue maturation with this prosthesis in situ (Fig 29).

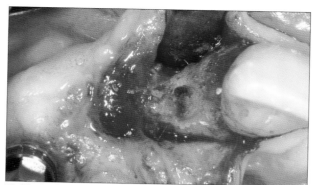

Fig 25   Implant-bed preparation at site 12.

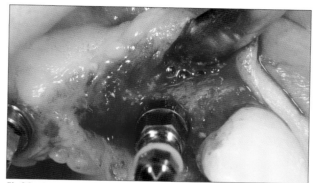

Fig 26   A narrow-neck implant was placed at the site of the lateral incisor.

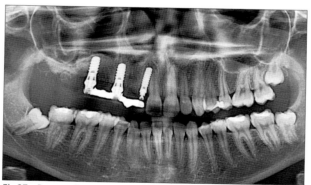

Fig 27   Panoramic radiograph demonstrating that the implants were correctly positioned under the provisional prosthesis.

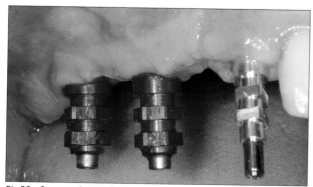

Fig 28   Screw-on impression caps for the open-tray impression.

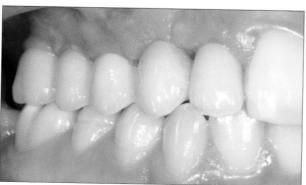

Fig 29   Lateral view of the provisional fixed prosthesis, now supported by three implants.

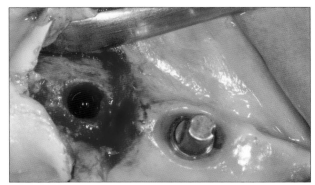

Fig 30   Osteotomes were used to prepare the second-molar site for implant placement.

The last surgical stage was performed to place an implant at the site of the second molar and to extract the impacted mandibular third molar. Due to the limited quantity and quality of bone at the site, the procedure was performed in accordance with Roccuzzo and Wilson (2009). Initial drilling was confined to using a 2.0-mm round bur at 680 rpm to facilitate the use of osteotomes in the sites. The osteotomy sites were prepared with Straumann osteotomes for sinus floor elevation (Straumann, Basel, Switzerland). Instruments of increasing diameters were gently tapped with a mallet to compress bone in an apicolateral direction. Further drilling was performed only when there was very strong resistance to the osteotome (Fig 30). A screw tap was not used. A chemically modified titanium implant (Standard Plus RN SLActive®, diameter 4.1 mm, length, 8 mm; Straumann, Basel, Switzerland) was placed at a transmucosal level (Fig 31).

The definitive restoration consisted in a five-unit fixed partial denture with solid abutments tightened to the three posterior implants at 35 Ncm (Fig 32) plus a single crown delivered via a customized screw-retained zirconia abutment (CARES® CADCAM abutment; Straumann, Basel, Switzerland) to the anterior implant at the lateral-incisor site (Fig 33).

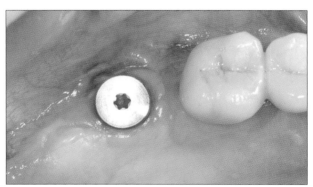

Fig 31   Healing status 6 weeks after placing the implant at site 17.

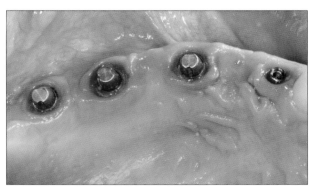

Fig 32   A five-unit fixed partial denture was cemented to three 4-mm solid abutments.

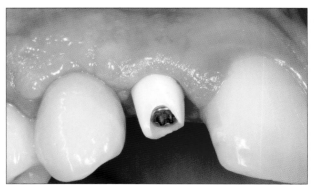

Fig 33   At the lateral-incisor site, a zirconia abutment was selected to support a single crown.

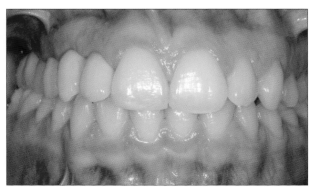

Fig 34   Frontal view of the final restorations in occlusion.

The panoramic radiograph from November 2011 confirmed that the peri-implant bone levels were stable (Fig 35).

The last clinical view was obtained more than 5 years after the car accident in January 2012. Again, the soft-tissue contours were stable and showed no signs of inflammation or significant recessions (Fig 36).

Periapical radiographs from July 2013 confirmed stable peri-implant bone levels (Fig 37).

Acknowledgments

Endodontic and restorative procedures
Dr. Giorgio Tessore – Turin, Italy

Laboratory procedures
Francesco Cataldi, Master Dental Technician – Turin, Italy

Professional maintenance
Silvia Gherlone, Registered Dental Hygienist – Turin, Italy

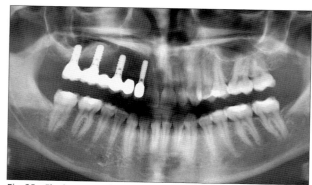

Fig 35   Final panoramic radiograph. Stable peri-implant bone levels around both the five-unit fixed partial denture and the implant-supported single crown.

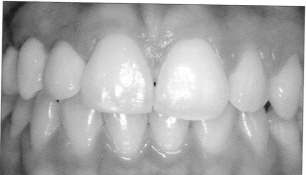

Fig 36   More than 5 years after the car accident, a frontal view in occlusion showed stable peri-implant soft tissues.

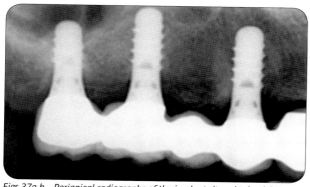

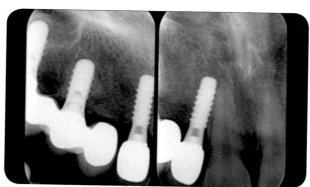

Figs 37a-b   Periapical radiographs of the implant sites obtained 6.5 years after treatment.

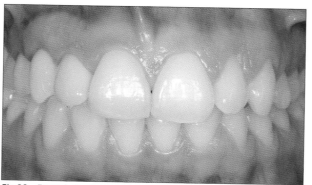

Fig 38   Frontal view in occlusion. Good stability of the peri-implant soft tissues was noted even 6.5 years after implant treatment.

6.7   Shell Technique for Horizontal and Vertical Maxillary Bone Augmentation in a Partially Edentulous Patient with Aggressive Periodontal Disease

Luca Cordaro

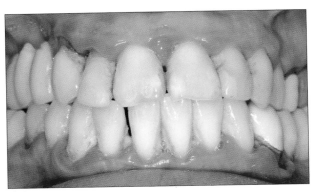

Fig 1a

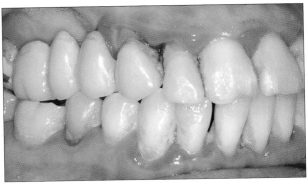

Fig 1b

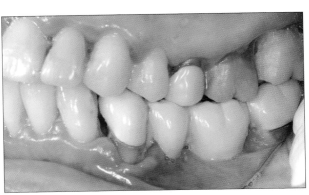

Fig 1c

A 46-year-old woman was referred for treatment whose main complaints were mobility of her fixed partial dentures (right maxilla and left mandible) and periodontal bleeding during function. She also reported having taken systemic antibiotics to treat recurrent swelling in the area of the upper left molars.

The patient had not seen a dentist for at least 2 years. She did not smoke and had no history of major systemic disease other than two minor orthopedic procedures some years back.

The first-visit examination revealed poor plaque control, tooth mobility, periodontal disease, and a residual dentition widely associated with deep periodontal pockets (Figs 1a-f).

Despite the obvious nature of her chronic periodontitis, the patient was not aware of having a pathological condition and reported that she had not previously been informed about the effects of plaque on periodontal tissues.

Figs 1a-f   Clinical views and panoramic radiograph at presentation. It was clear that the patient's plaque control was poor and that a diagnosis of advanced periodontal disease was imminent. A definitive treatment plan could not be proposed. In this kind of situation, any further treatment decisions should be preceded by periodontal treatment (including scaling and root planing) and extraction of any teeth that would be irrational to treat. Hygiene instructions and patient motivation are also mandatory. There should be no attempt to implement a definitive fixed rehabilitation before the periodontal disease is controlled. The occlusal views of both jaws demonstrate a great amount of calculus and plaque accumulation on the palatal and lingual sides of the dentition. The panoramic radiograph confirms the extent of bone resorption in the first and third quadrants. Signs of advanced periodontal breakdown were seen in all quadrants.

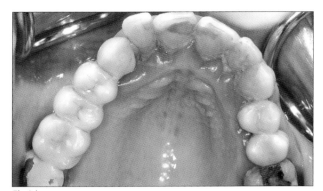

Fig 1d

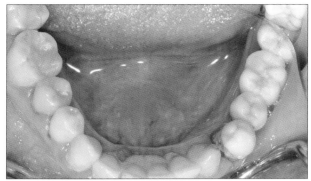

Fig 1e

An initial course of periodontal treatment was started, including the establishment of proper oral hygiene, patient motivation, scaling, and root planing. After removing the fixed partial dentures in the first and third quadrants due to their grade III mobility, all remaining tooth abutments distal to the upper right central incisor and the lower left canine were extracted.

Since the initial treatment phase is as important as the rehabilitation phase, this was the time to establish compliance and to convey to the patient an understanding of the chronic nature of her disease. There was a need for her to accept that supportive maintenance therapy would have to be provided continuously for the rest of her life.

Compliance had improved when the patient was reevaluated 3 months into the treatment. Plaque and bleeding scores were greatly improved. Beyond the removable partial denture for provisional use in the maxilla, the mobility of the residual dentition was back to normal (Figs 2a-c). The maxilla was found to require more periodontal treatment by surgical means and to accommodate residual molars whose prognosis was questionable.

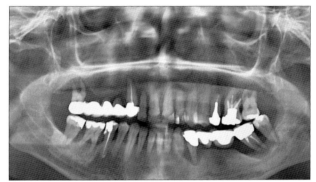

Fig 1f

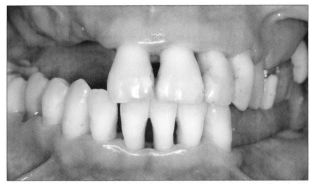

Figs 2a-c Clinical views after initial periodontal and extraction (teeth 17, 13, 12, 37, 34) treatment. Note the dramatic improvement in periodontal health and the clearly visible effects of alveolar bone resorption.

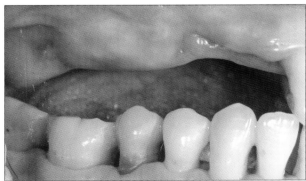

Fig 2b

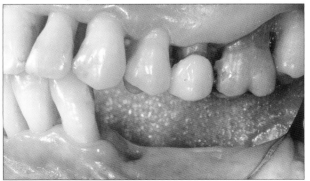

Fig 2c

Table 1   Treatment plan (M: tooth missing at presentation; MI: missing tooth and implant placement; EX: extraction; EXI: extraction and implant placement; IFDP: implant-supported fixed dental prosthesis).

Maxillary site	17	16	15	14	13	12	11	21	22	23	24	25	26	27
Extraction/implant	EX	MI	MI	M	EXI	EX							EXI	EX
Superstructure		IFDP	IFDP	IFDP	IFDP	IFDP						Crown	Crown	
Superstructure											IFDP	IFDP	IFDP	
Extraction/implant											EXI	M	MI	EX
Mandibular site	47	46	45	44	43	42	41	31	32	33	34	35	36	37

After discussing a prosthetic treatment plan with the patient, it was decided to restore all missing teeth in both arches back to the first molars, using implant-supported fixed partial dentures where needed and replacing the old crown restoration on the upper left second premolar.

Part of this plan was to insert three implants in the first quadrant (sites 16, 15, 13) for a five-unit prosthesis featuring a cantilever unit on tooth 12. Only one implant-supported crown was planned in the second quadrant, restoring the extracted first but not the second molar, besides the aforementioned tooth-supported crown for the second premolar.

The third quadrant was to be restored with a three-unit fixed partial denture supported by two implants at the sites of the first molar and first premolar. No prosthetic work was required in the fourth quadrant (Table 1).

Since a major bone defect was anticipated on extracting the upper right canine, it was proposed to go ahead with implant surgery in the three quadrants in the knowledge that staged bone reconstruction would be required in the first quadrant.

It was determined that the surgical treatment needs in preparation for implant placement would include resective periodontics to deal with a number of persistent deep pockets at the remaining upper dentition and a block graft for bone augmentation in the first quadrant.

Along with carrying out resective surgery in the maxillary arch, the upper first and second left molars were extracted because of deep pockets, mobility, and furcation involvement.

Bone augmentation in the first quadrant was conducted with conscious sedation under local anesthesia. A midcrestal incision was performed, extended to the sulcus of the adjacent central incisor, and terminated distally in only one vertical releasing incision at the site of the right third molar. Access to the ridge was created by wide subperiosteal dissection. A vertical and horizontal through-and-through defect with complete destruction of the bony ridge was evident along the sites of the lateral incisor, canine, and first premolar (Fig 3a).

Bone-block harvesting was started from the mandibular ramus and angle on the ipsilateral side. After harvesting and partial milling, the block was adapted and secured to the recipient site with two titanium lag screws to reconstruct the missing facial bone wall of the defect (Figs 3b-c). The residual defect was packed with autologous bone chips (obtained by milling part of the block) and bovine-bone grafting material (Fig 3d). Care was taken to achieve horizontal overcontouring of the defect. No membrane was used to cover the reconstruction.

The flap was released with appropriate periosteal incisions and sutured with horizontal mattress sutures and continuous sutures.

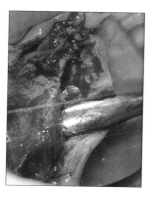

Fig 3a Flap elevation clearly revealed the through-and-through nature of this vertical and horizontal defect, which offered very adverse conditions for augmentation. The extent of the bone destruction was due to a periodontal lesion related to a canine preserved under a mobile fixed partial denture.

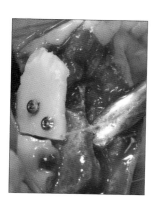

Fig 3b Lateral view of the block harvested from the mandibular ramus and secured to the recipient site with two titanium screws 1.5 mm in diameter. This block would ensure an adequate gain in horizontal dimension.

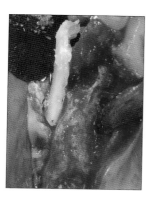

Fig 3c Occlusal view of the bone block in situ, illustrating the amount of particulate material that would be needed to fill the defect and complete the reconstruction.

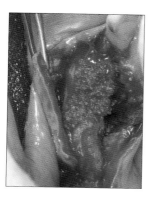

Fig 3d Part of the ramus-derived block was milled and mixed with bovine bone graft material at a 2 : 1 ratio, resulting in a particulate graft used to fill the residual defect underneath the mandibular block. A covering membrane was not used in this specific case.

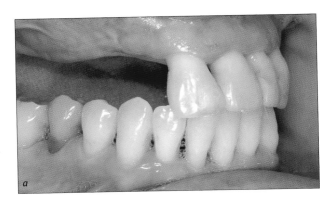

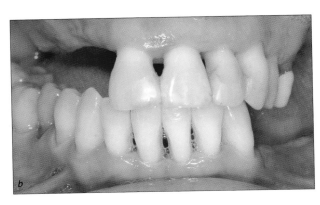

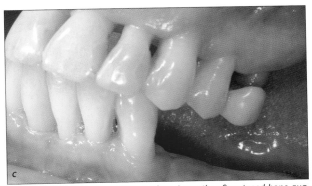

Observations made 4 months after the procedure included healing of the augmented region and the presence of adequate hard-tissue support to the soft tissues (Figs 4a-c). This was the time to work out the final plan for implant surgery. As careful evaluation of the interproximal space distal to the right central incisor confirmed a total lack of papilla even now that the probing depth was minimal, it was decided to place the mesial implant at the canine site and restore the lateral incisor with a cantilever unit.

Figs 4a-c   Intraoral views of the patient 4 months after staged bone augmentation. The clinical situation demonstrated that the time had come for implant placement: periodontal disease was under control, patient compliance had improved, and the outcome of bone reconstruction looked successful. Esthetic considerations of extensively receded papillae throughout the maxilla and long clinical crowns remained a major concern at this point.

Implant surgery was performed after 4 months of healing. A full-thickness flap was raised via a crestal incision to gain access to the reconstructed bone for removal of the screws that had been inserted for bone-block fixation. The bone was found to be nicely reconstructed (Figs 5a-b). Three tissue-level implants (Soft Tissue Level SLActive®, diameter 4.1 mm, Straumann, Basel, Switzerland) were placed for transmucosal healing at the sites of the first molar, second premolar, and canine (Figs 5c-d).

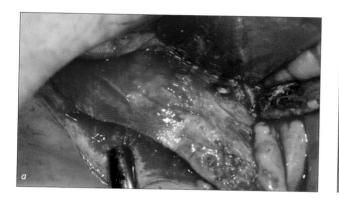
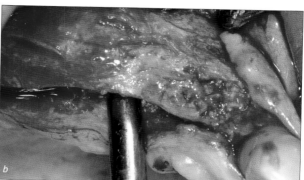
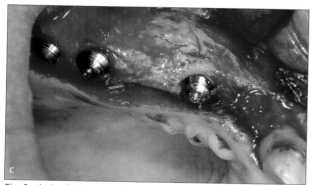
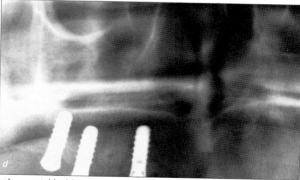

Figs 5a-d   Implant surgery. Access to the reconstructed crest was created through a crestal incision and a distal releasing incision. An effective outcome of reconstruction was clearly visible both from the lateral (a) and occlusal (b) view at this point. Implants were placed at the sites of the first molar, second premolar, and canine—planning a cantilever unit at the lateral-incisor site (c). Radiograph of the first-quadrant implants before loading (d).

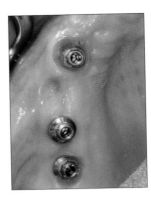

Fig 6   Final soft-tissue situation in the reconstructed area. The soft tissues were healthy and had adequate hard-tissue support by that time. This picture was taken at the time of delivering the definitive fixed partial denture. Patience compliance was also confirmed at this point. The major goals of this complex treatment plan had been achieved.

During the uneventful healing of the implant sites, the remaining implants were placed in the second and third quadrants, the latter requiring a GBR procedure simultaneously with implant placement to deal with a moderate horizontal defect at the first-premolar site. The final prosthetic stages were initiated 8 weeks after implant surgery in the first quadrant.

In accordance with the treatment plan, the patient was provided with five-unit fixed partial denture retained by screws on the right side of the maxilla. Both the soft-tissue situation in the reconstructed area and patient compliance had reached a favorable level by that time (Fig 6). Horizontal bony support of the soft tissues was confirmed. The other edentulous spaces were restored with two single crowns supported by one natural tooth and one implant on the left side of the maxilla and a three-unit cemented prosthesis supported by implants at the first-premolar and first-molar sites on the left side of the mandible. The total duration of treatment—including the periodontal pretreatment steps—was 10 months.

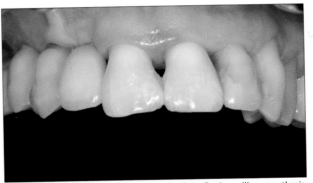

Figs 7a-c   Close-up views and radiograph of the final maxillary prosthesis, illustrating the outcome of treatment a few days after delivery. Advanced resorption of periodontal support by hard and soft tissues was visible along the residual natural dentition. The functional and esthetic outcome in the maxilla was to the patient's satisfaction. The close-up view of the reconstructed area illustrates acceptable esthetics with healthy periodontal and peri-implant soft tissues. The radiographic view demonstrates successful treatment.

The images in Figures 7a-c show the final maxillary prosthesis a few days after delivery. Rehabilitating the right side of the maxilla in this patient was the most demanding part of a complex and meticulous treatment plan. Acceptable function and esthetics had been achieved, considering the initially advanced resorption of periodontal support to the natural dentition. The patient was very happy with the achieved outcome and declined further treatment to replace the old composite restorations across her residual dentition.

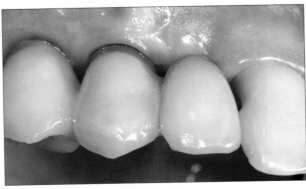

Fig 7b

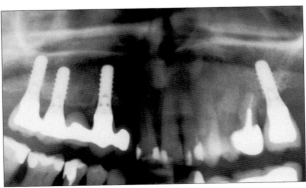

Fig 7c

Restorative treatment was followed by instituting a supportive maintenance protocol with professional oral-hygiene sessions every 4 months. Given the absence of any additional risk factors like smoking or diabetes, it was reasonable to expect a good prognosis.

Good stability of the outcome was observed 4 years after the end of active periodontal and restorative treatment, confirming that patient compliance was good and disease progression effectively under control (Figs 8a-b). No more active treatment had taken place by that time.

Implementing a fixed implant-supported restoration in situations of extensive tooth loss due to periodontal diseases will facilitate the maintenance of adequate oral hygiene compared to a removable partial denture. Every attempt should be made to deliver a fixed restoration, including staged reconstruction of the atrophic jawbone if necessary. Ideal augmentation techniques should be selected to effectively deal with specific defect types and dimensions. The present case, characterized by an extensive vertical defect, was managed by a block graft harvested from the mandibular ramus in combination with a particulated mixture of bone substitute and autologous chips. The reconstruction was successful and allowed the implants needed for the planned superstructures to be safely and effectively inserted.

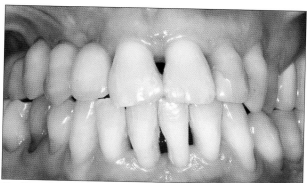

Figs 8a-c State of the reconstruction at the 4-year follow-up, including clinical views that illustrate good stability of the soft tissues and a radiograph that confirms long-term stability of the bone reconstruction.

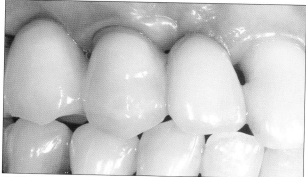

Fig 8b

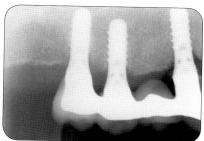

Fig 8c

6.8 Horizontal Augmentation with Iliac Bone Grafts in the Treatment of Non-Syndromic Oligodontia

D. Weingart

A 20-year-old woman was referred for implant therapy in 2004. Her medical history revealed no significant findings, and neither did she smoke nor take any medications. An extraoral examination revealed no abnormalities of the skin, hair or nails. The intraoral examination revealed only 11 permanent teeth clinically. These were normal in shape, size, and color.

In addition, eight retained deciduous teeth (53, 62, 63, 71, 72, 73, 81, 82) were present. No abnormalities were detected during the general examination. The family history revealed that the patient's father and two sisters were on record with similar conditions. The clinical examination revealed a thick gingival biotype. No recession of the attached gingiva was noted, but the retained deciduous teeth were mobile and unsightly. As a syndrome had not been diagnosed, the case was categorized as non-syndromic oligodontia. A panoramic radiograph was obtained which, disregarding third molars, revealed agenesis of 17 permanent teeth (18, 13, 12, 22, 23, 27, 37, 35 – 31, 41 – 44, 47). The retained deciduous teeth were affected by generalized root resorption.

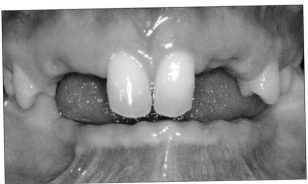

Fig 1   Frontal view of prospective implant areas.

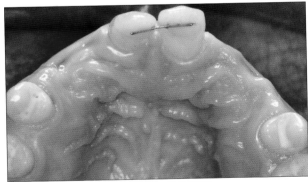

Fig 2   Occlusal view of prospective implant areas.

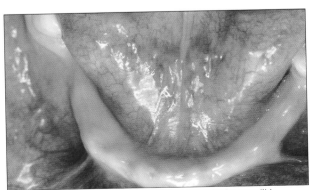

Fig 3   Occlusal view of prospective implant areas in the mandible.

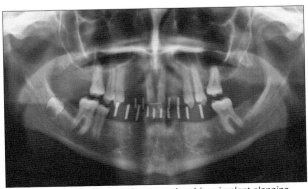

Fig 4   Panoramic radiograph for restoration-driven implant planning.

Treatment plan

After discussing treatment options with the patient, it was agreed to proceed with the following plan:

- Extraction of the retained deciduous teeth
- Horizontal augmentation at sites 13, 12, 22, 23, 36–45 with autologous bone grafts from the iliac crest under general anesthesia
- Implant placement at sites 14, 13, 22, 23, 35 – 32, 42 – 45
- Reopening procedure and initiation of soft-tissue conditioning by means of a provisional implant-supported fixed prosthesis
- Final delivery of a metal-ceramic fixed prosthesis 4 months later
- Postsurgical maintenance, including reinforcement of oral hygiene and ultrasonic debridement, every 6 months

The patient gave her informed consent. Treatment was started by extracting the retained deciduous teeth atraumatically without flap elevation. The extraction sockets were debrided and fitted with collagen plugs for hemostasis. Subsequently the patient was provided with a removable partial denture that would allow the extraction sites to heal with formation of an increased band of keratinized mucosa (Figs 1 to 3).

Surgery for bone augmentation was preceded by restoration-driven implant planning (Fig 4).

A waiting period of 12 weeks ensued after the extraction procedure. Subsequently the procedure of bone augmentation with corticocancellous grafts from the iliac crest was conducted under general anesthesia. The first step was to perform a midcrestal incision along the edentulous ridge and one vertical releasing incision (Fig 5).

On identifying the mental foramens and the mental nerve, the periosteum was reflected and a round bur applied to smooth the occlusal aspect of the alveolar crest. Then a prepared surgical stent was placed to assess the three-dimensional needs for bone augmentation at the planned implant sites. Corticocancellous bone was harvested from the iliac crest, adapted to the alveolar bone, and secured with titanium lag screws to ensure close contact. In addition, particulated bone was placed around the block grafts for ridge contouring (Fig 6).

The augmented sites were then covered with collagen membranes (Bio-Gide®; Geistlich Biomaterials, Wolhusen, Switzerland). After a periosteal incision, the soft tissues were mobilized to ensure tension-free wound closure in the mandible. Both a block graft and particulated autologous bone were used for horizontal

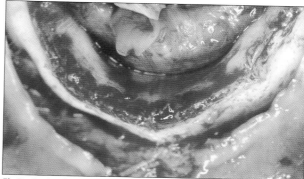
Fig 5   Occlusal view of the incision design in the mandible.

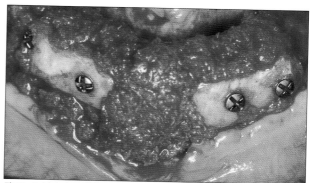
Fig 6   Labial view of the augmentation site in the mandible.

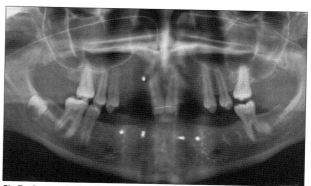
Fig 7   Postsurgical radiograph.

augmentation on the right side of the anterior maxilla, while the defect morphology at sites 22 and 23 indicated the use of particulated bone only. As in the mandible, the augmented areas were covered with a collagen membrane (Fig 7).

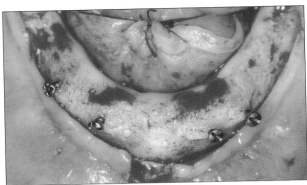

Fig 8   Occlusal view of the augmented mandible.

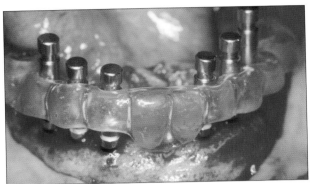

Fig 9   Labial view of the surgical stent in the mandible.

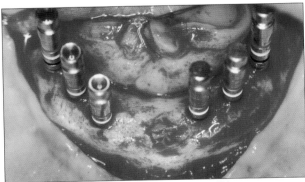

Fig 10   Labial view of the implant sites in the mandible.

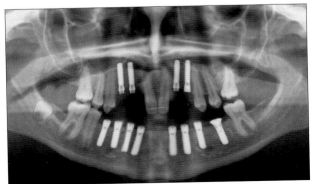

Fig 11   Panoramic radiograph obtained after implant surgery.

After 6 months of healing, implant surgery was performed under general anesthesia. This procedure was initiated via a midcrestal incision along the previous incision line (Fig 8).

After elevating a full-thickness flap and carefully removing the lag screws, implants were inserted (sites 13, 14, 22, 23, 35 – 32, 42 – 45) with the aid of a surgical stent (Figs 9 and 10).

Soft tissue-level implants were used at all sites in this patient (Standard Plus NN SLA®, diameter 3.3 mm, lengths 10 and 12 mm; at site 36, Standard Plus RN SLA®, diameter 4.1 mm, length 10 mm; Straumann, Basel, Switzerland). Additional local grafting was performed with bone particles collected from the implant beds via a bone trap. After covering the augmented sites with collagen membranes (Bio-Gide®; Geistlich, Wolhusen, Switzerland), primary wound closure was achieved for submerged healing (Fig 11). Postsurgically, the edentulous areas of the existing removable partial dentures were modified to avoid direct contact with the wound area.

After 3 months of uneventful healing, all implants were uncovered via a minor incision but without flap elevation to facilitate healing (Fig 12).

Within 1 week, a provisional restoration was inserted, using titanium copings and acrylic, to initiate the soft-tissue conditioning phase. Good healing of the peri-implant soft tissues was noted, resulting in an architecture similar to the one of healthy gingival tissue around natural teeth. Metal-ceramic fixed prostheses were delivered as final restorations (Figs 13 to 15). The patient was recalled every 6 months for maintenance therapy.

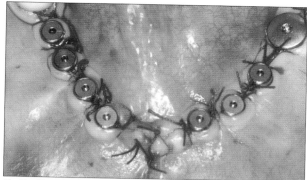

Fig 12   Situation in the mandible after second-stage surgery.

Discussion

Missing teeth may cause significant esthetic, functional, and psychological problems in young patients especially if anterior jaw segments are involved (Gorlin and coworkers 1975; Stewart and coworkers 1982). Relevant developmental anomalies have been classified as "oligodontia" when at least six teeth other than third molars are congenitally missing versus "hypodontia" with agenesis of less than six teeth (Çakur and coworkers 2006). Cases of oligodontia usually form part of congenital syndromes that affect several organ systems and may be associated with various genetic syndromes, ectodermal dysplasia being one example (Çakur and coworkers 2006). Early diagnosis of, and treatment planning for, patients with "syndromic oligodontia" is facilitated by typical abnormalities of the skin, nails, eyes, ears, and skeleton. Rare cases of "non-syndromic oligodontia" are, however, known to exist as well. While the etiology of oligodontia is not fully understood, the fact that genetic factors seem to play a major part stresses the relevance of family histories (Çakur and coworkers 2006). Our patient shared her clinical symptoms with both her father and her two sisters.

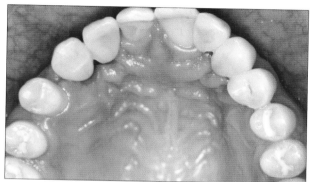

Fig 13   Occlusal view of the final prosthesis in the maxilla.

Possibilities of oral rehabilitation with implant-supported prostheses have expanded range of treatment options in patients with varying degrees of edentulism (Weingart and ten Bruggenkate 2000). Any success of implant treatment will depend, to a large extent, on the quality and the quantity of bone at the recipient site. Long-term stability and esthetics can be achieved by adequate bone grafting procedures, allowing for predictable treatment outcomes even in initially deficient bone situations (Weingart and ten Bruggenkate 2000).

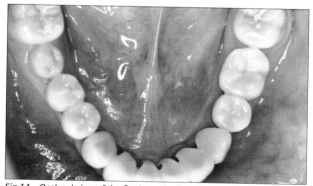

Fig 14   Occlusal view of the final prosthesis in the mandible.

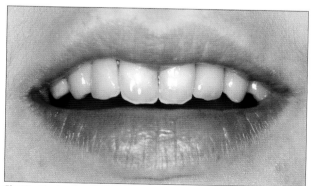

Fig 15   Final restoration and lip line.

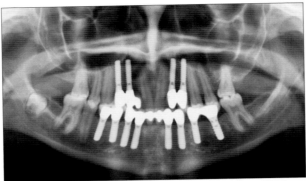

Fig 16   Panoramic radiograph 1 year after prosthetic delivery (2005).

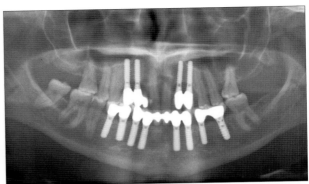

Fig 17   Panoramic radiograph 7 years after prosthetic delivery (2012).

Autologous grafting is the gold standard for bone regeneration. The case here presented has been managed by combined use of block grafts and bone particles for horizontal augmentation with additional coverage by a resorbable collagen barrier membrane (Bio-Gide®; Geistlich, Wolhusen, Switzerland) for guided bone regeneration. Bone particles offer several benefits for horizontal augmentation: they (a) can be readily adapted to any irregular elements of defect morphology; (b) offer ideal porosity to promote migration of osteogenic cells; (c) are capable of releasing osteoinductive growth factors; and (d) create a natural osteoconductive surface for cell at-

tachment and growth (Bonewald 2011; Miron and coworkers 2011). That said, the use of a barrier membrane is warranted as bone particles may be unstable and get displaced from the defect during healing. This approach was successfully utilized in the case here presented to restore the horizontal thickness and vertical height of the buccal bone wall; both factors are keys to esthetic and functional success. Both panoramic radiographs obtained after 1 year and 7 years reveal good stability of the peri-implant bone levels, meeting an essential requirement for long-term function and esthetics (Figs 16 and 17).

6.9 Bilateral Horizontal Ridge Augmentation with Block Bone Grafts Using a Piezo-electric Device for Fixed Implant Restoration

Y.-D. Kwon

A woman in her mid-fifties was referred by a dental student for dental implant placement. Both posterior segments of the mandible had been edentulous for more than 4 years, the only residual tooth being the right lower first premolar (Fig 1a). The patient had used a removable partial denture but was not entirely satisfied with its function.

The clinical examination revealed a sharp edentulous ridge in both posterior segments of the mandible, and the patient was told that it would not be possible to insert implants into this thin edentulous ridge without significant augmentation of the alveolar ridge.

Her medical history revealed no significant findings and no underlying disease that might have complicated surgical procedures. During the presurgical examination, the patient reported that she was a little apprehensive about bone grafting. After being informed about the surgical procedures and potential postoperative complications, she accepted the proposed surgical plan of bone grafting and subsequent placement of implants.

The preoperative orthopantomogram (Fig 1b) confirmed that all mandibular premolars and molars other than tooth 34 were missing.

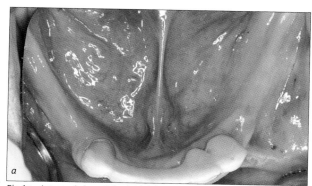

Fig 1a   Intraoral view of the initial situation.

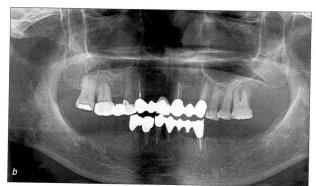

Fig 1b   Orthopantomogram of the initial situation.

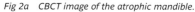

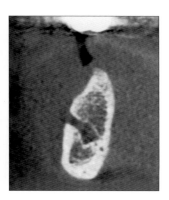

Fig 2a   CBCT image of the atrophic mandible.

Fig 2b   CBCT image of the sharp and atrophic alveolar ridge at site 45.

A cone-beam computed tomography (CBCT) scan was obtained to visualize the edentulous ridge and nearby anatomical structures (Figs 2a-b). Tooth 26 was to be extracted after consulting a periodontologist for an opinion about its prognosis. There was no need for vertical augmentation in this patient because the height of the alveolar ridge was quite well preserved based on the clinical and radiographic findings.

Treatment plan
- Extraction of tooth 26
- Block bone graft from the posterior mandible on both mandibular premolar and molar regions
- Metal-ceramic fixed prosthesis for the mandibular anterior segment
- Three implants for the right posterior segment of the mandible
- Two implants for the left posterior segment of the mandible
- Metal-ceramic bridges

This plan was agreed on after several treatment options had been discussed with the patient. She was informed of potential risks and gave her written informed consent.

Surgical procedures
An inferior alveolar nerve block was carried out and a full-thickness mucoperiosteal flap elevated from the distal surface of a canine to the ascending ramus region. A small vertical incision was performed at the mesial line angle of the canine (Figs 3a-b). The distal part of the incision was flared (Fig 3a) in order to expose the anterior ascending ramus, enabling access to the region where a bone block could be harvested. While a second surgical site is normally mandatory to harvest a bone block, this specific case could be managed with a single incision to cover both the donor and the recipient site.

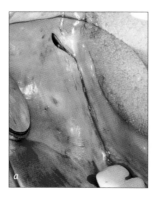
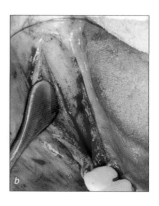

Figs 3a-b   A full-thickness mucoperiosteal flap was raised at the recipient site.

Table 1   Comparison between the two major intraoral donor sites for bone-block grafts.

Sites	Advantages	Disadvantages
Chin	Easy access More bone volume Easy harvesting of blocks and chips	Wound dehiscence Pulp damage (potentially permanent) Sensory disturbances
Posterior mandible	Familiarity (ramus/third-molar surgery) Uncomplicated healing Low rate of sequelae	Less bone volume Limited visibility Proximity to inferior alveolar nerve

Among intraoral donor sites, the posterior mandible—including the anterior ramus—and the mandibular chin are the most widely utilized sources for bone-block grafts. Both sites have their strengths and weaknesses.

Both donor sites are capable of offering enough bone for most reconstructions of partially edentulous ridges in conjunction with bone fillers. Which of both should be used will depend on a number of factors, including the location of the defect and the surgeon's preference.

Options available to perform the osteotomy include rotary instruments and piezoelectric devices. The latter are used more commonly, as they can minimize soft-tissue injuries and patient anxiety (Fig 4). Surgical vision may be more limited, and soft-tissue protection is more demanding, in the posterior mandible than in the chin area.

It is always crucial to ensure that all cortical margins of the bone block are fully cut, an exception being the inferior osteotomy line connecting two vertical osteotomies. In this situation, each osteotomy line may pass the point where the lines meet to ensure complete separation of the block (Fig 5).

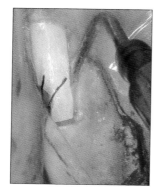

Fig 4   Osteotomy performed in the anterior ramus area. A piezoelectric device was used for easier and more efficient bone cutting.

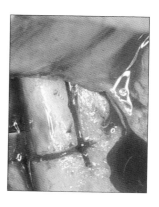

Fig 5   An osteotomy line passing the point where the lines meet. An inferior osteotomy can be performed using various working tips on the piezoelectric device.

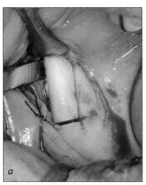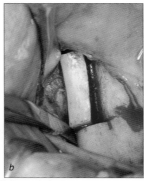

Figs 6a-b   A cortical graft can be readily harvested using an osteotome.

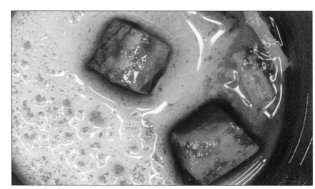

Fig 7   A block graft may be divided to optimize its stability on the recipient site.

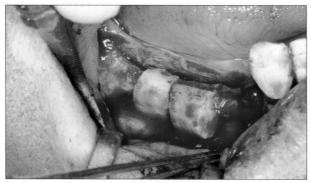

Fig 8   The grafts were trimmed and adapted.

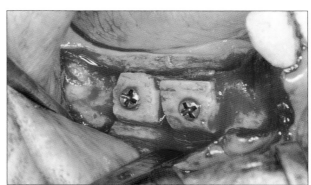

Fig 9   Titanium screws (2.0 × 10 mm; Jeil Corporation, Seoul, South Korea) were used to fixate the grafts in accordance with the lag-screw principle. After elevating the lingual flap, a periosteal elevator was inserted to protect the periosteum and allow a drill to penetrate the lingual cortical plate.

Using the curved blade on the piezoelectric device, which can access the lateral side of the posterior mandible and anterior ramus, a gutter can be made on the lateral side of the posterior mandible, connecting two vertical osteotomies. The gutter remains in the cortical bone and does not have to enter the medullary bone. The block of bone can be readily separated by light tapping on the osteotomy lines with a osteotome mallet (Figs 6a-b).

Blocks can be adjusted to fit the surface architecture of their intended recipient areas (Fig 7). They should provide as much contact as possible for optimal stability (Fig 8). Blocks from the posterior mandible have an inverted-J shape well suited for adaptation to horizontal bone defects in mandibular molar areas. Blocks may be divided for fixation, maximizing the contact area with the recipient site and allowing separate fixation to future implant sites.

One screw is normally sufficient to secure a block graft. For maximum graft stability, it should engage three cortical layers, including the block graft and the buccal and cortical plates of the recipient site. Also, the lag-screw principle should be applied to ensure tight contact between the graft and recipient site.

To effectively preserve the augmented volume, it is beneficial to cover the autologous bone block with deproteinized bovine bone substitute and/or a barrier membrane (Figs 10 to 12) (Maiorana and coworkers 2005; von Arx and Buser 2006).

Offering additional protection may significantly increase the volume stability of a bone-block graft. Tension-free primary closure was achieved via a periosteal releasing incision. The horizontal bone gain attained was significant (Figs 13a-b and 14a-b).

The same procedure was carried out on the left side.

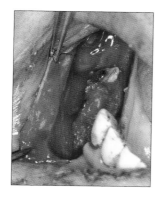

Fig 10 Deproteinized bovine bone chips were used to fill some voids between the grafts. Tension-free wound closure was achieved via a periosteal releasing incision.

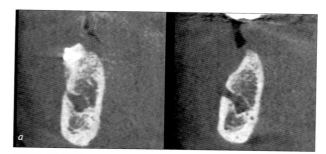

Fig 11 Double-layered application of a collagen membrane to protect the graft.

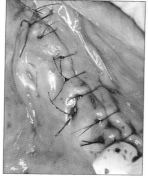

Fig 12 Soft-tissue closure with 4-0 monofilament sutures.

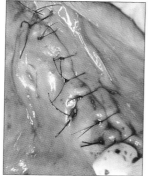

Figs 13a-b (a) Coronal and (b) cross-sectional views of the pre- and post-surgical CBCT images. Sizeable amount of horizontal bone augmentation.

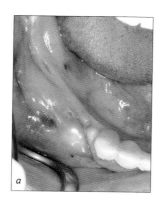

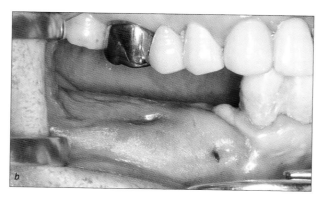

Figs 14a-b Clinical views obtained 4 months after bone-block grafting. A noticeable gain in bone width had been achieved in the right posterior segment of the mandible.

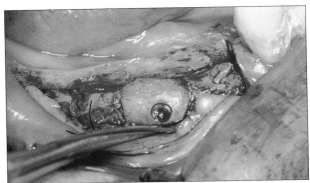

Fig 15   Elevation of a full-thickness flap for implant placement. On removing the fixation screws, the fully healed block graft was exposed to view.

Four months after the grafting procedure, the bone block was fully integrated at the recipient site (Figs 15 and 18). Three implants (Tissue Level, diameter 4.1 mm, length 12 mm, at site 44; Tissue Level, diameter 4.8 mm, length 10 mm, at site 46; Tissue Level, diameter 4.1 mm, length 8 mm, at site 47; all three Straumann, Basel, Switzerland) were placed in the right posterior segment of the mandible (Fig 16) and two implants (Tissue Level, diameter 4.1 mm, length 10 mm, at site 34; Tissue Level, diameter 4.1 mm, length 8 mm, at site 36; both Straumann) in the left segment (Fig 19).

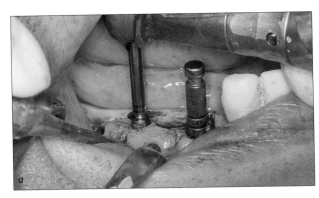
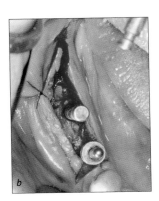
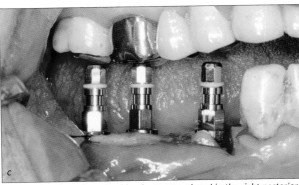
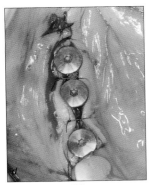

Figs 16a-d   Three tissue-level implants were placed in the right posterior segment of the mandible.

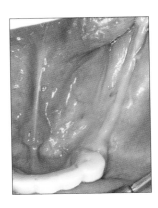

Fig 17   Clinical view of the left posterior segment 4 months after bone-block grafting.

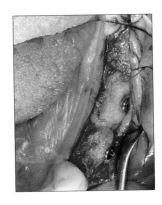

Fig 18   Successful horizontal augmentation and ideal integration of the block grafts.

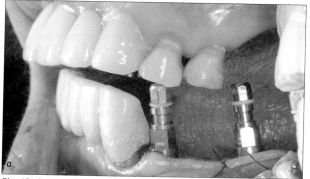
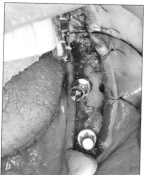

Figs 19a-b   Two tissue-level implants were placed in the left posterior segment.

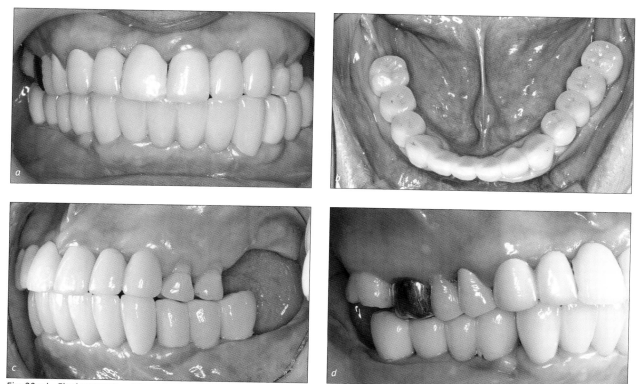

Figs 20a-d   Final restorations. The patient was happy with the chewing function of her new restoration.

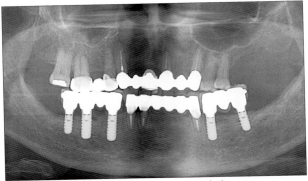

Fig 21   Orthopantomogram 3 months postoperatively.

Restoration and follow-up

Metal-ceramic bridges were delivered. She was happy with the chewing function of her new restoration.

When the patient was seen for a follow-up examination 2.5 years after delivering the final restorations, she revealed no signs of complications. The stability of the marginal bone levels was radiographically verified and considered good.

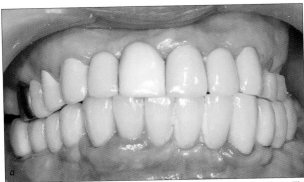

Figs 22a-c   Situation 2.5 years after delivery of the final restorations. The peri-implant tissues appeared stable compared to their status immediately after delivery.

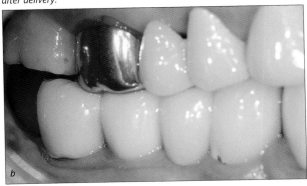

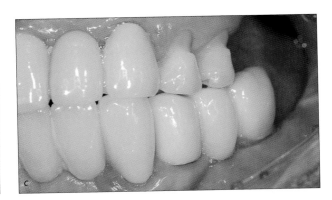

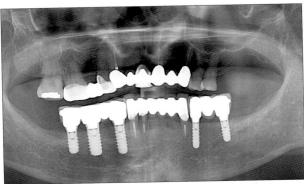

Fig 23   Orthopantomogram 2.5 years after delivery of the final restorations. The bone levels surrounding the implants appeared stable. Peri-implant bone loss was minimal.

6.10 Iliac and Calvarial Bone Blocks for Onlay Grafting of a Severely Resorbed Edentulous Maxilla

M. Chiapasco, P. Casentini

A 45-year-old woman with a completely edentulous maxilla was referred to evaluate the possibility of rehabilitation with an implant-supported prosthesis. This patient was healthy and a non-smoker. She had been wearing a maxillary complete denture opposing a natural mandibular dentition since her twenties. This situation had resulted in progressive resorption of the alveolar ridge, repeatedly creating a need for relining the denture. Twenty years later, despite multiple adaptations and the use of "glues," the denture was unstable and causing the patient psychological and functional discomfort.

A clinical and radiographic examination was performed at the consultation appointment, which revealed that the maxillary alveolar ridge was completely resorbed, with flattening of the palatal vault and distinct reduction of the buccal sulcus. Moreover, this total bone loss along the alveolar ridge had altered the intermaxillary vertical and horizontal relationships to a relevant degree of maxillary retrusion and an increased interarch distance (Figs 1 to 3). Also, the existing lack of hard tissue had compromised support to the lip and the perioral soft tissues, as reflected by an increase in perioral wrinkles and an "elderly" facial profile (Fig 4). It was evident that implants could not possibly be placed in this situation. A complex surgical reconstruction of the entire maxilla was unavoidable.

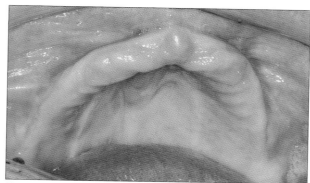

Figs 1 to 3   Initial clinical and radiographic views of the edentulous maxilla with severe atrophy. Given the extreme alveolar bone loss, it was impossible to place implants in this situation.

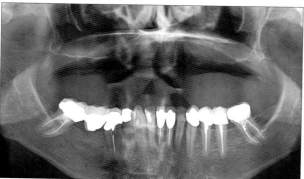

Fig 2

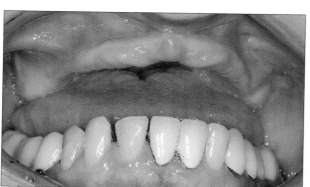

Fig 3

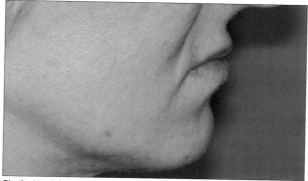

Fig 4   Hard-tissue loss had compromised support to the lip and perioral soft tissues.

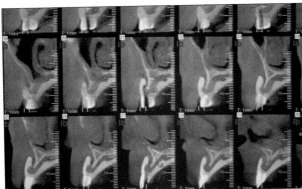 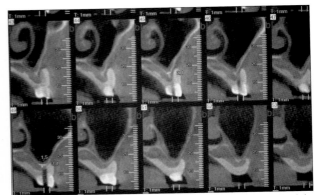

Figs 5 and 6   CT images before surgery with the patient wearing a radiopaque diagnostic template. The alveolar ridge was extremely resorbed and the residual bone did not have enough volume to allow for ideally positioned crowns.

Plaster casts were obtained to optimize the results from a surgical and prosthetic viewpoint, creating a diagnostic wax-up with ideal tooth positions without regard to the residual bone conditions. Computed tomography (CT) scans with the patient wearing a radiopaque template derived from the wax-up confirmed both that the posterior and anterior ridge segments were severely resorbed and that both maxillary sinuses were expanded. It was impossible to place implants in this situation (Figs 5 and 6).

Based on this clinical and radiographic evaluation, the case fell into the "complex" category of the SAC classification. Risk factors included (a) a total absence of residual alveolar bone associated with relevant sinus expansion, rendering implant insertion impossible; (b) an adverse intermaxillary relationship, rendering prosthetic rehabilitation complex; (c) a need to perform horizontal and vertical augmentation with autologous onlay grafts and sinus

floor elevation both bilaterally in the posterior segments and in the anterior segment of the maxilla; (d) a need for soft-tissue reconstruction following bone reconstruction; and (e) the need for complex restorative procedures.

A surgical plan was developed that included the use of autologous corticocancellous block grafts for vertical and horizontal augmentation of the edentulous maxilla and bilateral grafts for sinus floor elevation. Given the volume of augmentation required, the indication for bone harvesting was to exploit both the anterior ilium and the calvarium (right parietal bone). Eight implants (sites 16, 15, 14, 11, 21, 23, 24, 26) designed to support a fixed prosthesis were to be inserted in a second surgical stage 4 to 5 months after bone reconstruction.

The patient gave her informed consent to this treatment plan.

Reconstructive surgery

Surgery was conducted under general anesthesia by nasotracheal intubation. The first step was to perform a parasagittal incision in the parietal region down to the pericranium, which was then exposed by blunt dissection. Two pieces of the pericranium were harvested to cover the bone grafts late in the reconstructive procedure. Subsequently, three pieces of cortical bone from the outer cortex of the parietal bone were marked with fissure burs and removed with curved chisels, taking extreme care to avoid the sagittal sinus, not to expose the dura mater, or penetrate the brain, and to ensure that the inner cortex remained intact (Fig 7). After achieving hemostasis by applying bone wax, the surgical access was closed at the subcutaneous (resorbable 3-0 suture) and cutaneous (3-0 nylon suture) levels in two layers.

A second incision was performed along the anterior iliac crest, starting one centimeter behind the anterior iliac spine and exposing the iliac bone to allow harvesting from the medial side of the anterior iliac crest. This route was taken to avoid detaching muscles in the lateral thigh area and to reduce postoperative morbidity. The harvesting procedure included a corticocancellous block about 8 centimeters in length (Figs 8 and 9) and cancellous bone collected with a curette.

The iliac harvesting procedure was completed by placing a drain and closing the surgical access with multiple suture layers (periosteal, subcutaneous, cutaneous), using the same suture materials as previously on the skull.

Surgical access to the maxilla was established via a midcrestal incision extending from the left to the right maxillary tuberosity, supplemented by a vertical releasing incision at the midline to improve access to the bone. A mucoperiosteal full-thickness flap was elevated and the residual maxillary bone exposed on both the buccal and palatal aspects.

The first part of the surgical procedure was to elevate both sinus floors. Both sinuses were entered by creating osteotomies into the lateral sinus walls with round diamond burs attached to a straight low-speed handpiece and by elevating the Schneiderian membrane along with the lateral wall segments. The space created in the inferior part of either sinus was packed with autologous bone chips from the ilium, including both the cancellous component and some cortical bone particulated with a bone microtome.

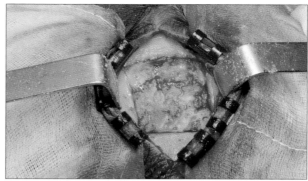

Figs 7 to 9 Given the significant volume of the planned reconstruction, bone was harvested both from the calvarium (Fig 7) and from the anterior iliac crest (Figs 8 and 9).

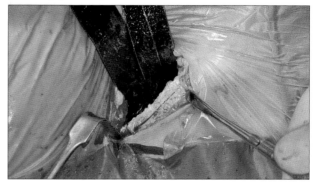

Fig 8

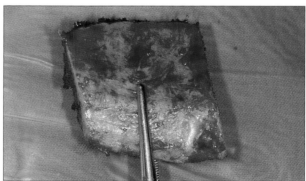

Fig 9

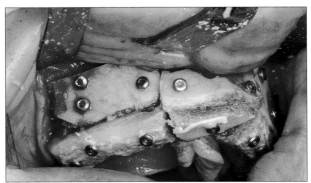

Figs 10 and 11 Three-dimensional reconstruction of the maxilla by means of bilateral sinus grafting and horizontal and vertical bone grafts fixated with titanium microscrews.

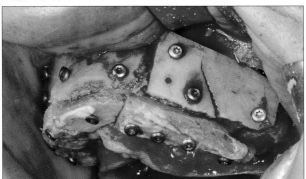

Fig 11

The bone block harvested from the ilium was separated into four pieces that were used, together with the calvarial segments, to reconstruct the severely resorbed maxilla both vertically and horizontally. The aim of this reconstruction was twofold: to increase the existing bone volume for the second-stage implant procedure and to restore appropriate intermaxillary relationships in the vertical, anteroposterior, and transversal dimensions. The bone blocks were rigidly stabilized with titanium microscrews (diameter: 1.5 mm). Any residual gaps between the bone blocks or between these and the recipient sites were densely packed with particulated autologous bone chips, eliminating any voids that might compromise the integration of the graft and improving the contour of the reconstructed area (Figs 10 to 12). Strips of pericranium were used to cover the bone grafts in an effort to minimize the risk of graft exposure in the event of wound dehiscence (Fig 13).

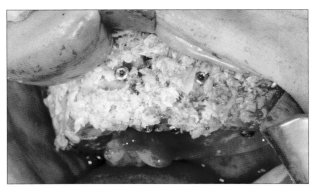

Figs 12 and 13 All voids between the autologous bone materials were filled with particulated bone and covered with autologous pericranium.

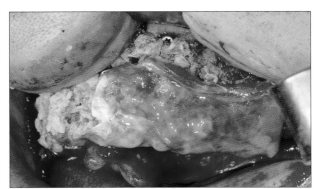

Fig 13

Releasing incisions of periosteum were performed in order to achieve a tension-free closure of the flap over the pericranium strips. 4-0 silk sutures were used (Fig 14).

Postoperative instructions included antibiotics for 1 week and chlorhexidine digluconate mouth rinses for two weeks.

Postoperative recovery was uneventful. The patient only experienced facial swelling for 1 week and some pain for 2 weeks.

The postoperative clinical and radiographic follow-up examinations revealed an appropriate bone gain, successful correction of intermaxillary relationships, and a noticeably improved facial profile resulting from enhanced support of the perioral soft tissues (Figs 15 and 16).

During the first postoperative month, the patient was not allowed to wear a removable prosthesis in the reconstructed area to avoid any problems with bone-graft integration and to minimize the risk of wound dehiscence/bone-graft exposure. After that time, she wore a softly relined removable denture without flanges (until implant surgery 5 months later).

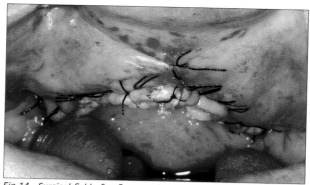

Fig 14   Surgical field after flap suturing at the end of the reconstructive procedure.

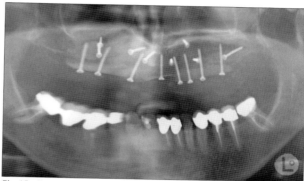

Fig 15   Panoramic radiograph obtained after the reconstructive procedure. Distinct bone gain.

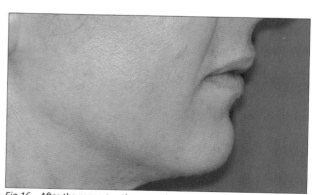

Fig 16   After the reconstructive procedure. Due to the soft-tissue support provided by the bone grafts, the patient's facial profile had clearly improved even in the absence of a prosthesis.

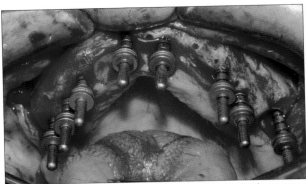

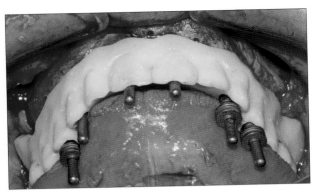

Figs 17 to 20   The situation 5 months later was ideal for implant surgery. After flap elevation, eight 3.3-mm Bone Level implants were inserted with guidance from a prefabricated surgical template.

Fig 18

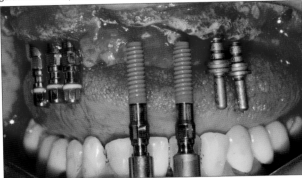

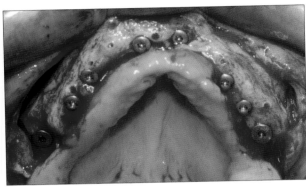

Fig 19

Fig 20

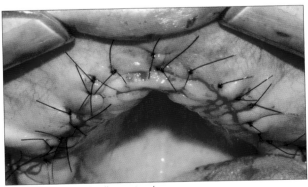

Implant surgery

Five months later, the previous incision was revisited and a mucoperiosteal flap raised to expose the reconstructed area. Integration of the graft was found to be excellent with no relevant bone loss.

Following the indications of a prefabricated surgical template, eight implants were placed in the reconstructed area (5 × Bone Level, diameter 3.3 mm, length 12 mm, at sites 14, 11, 21, 23, and 24; 1 × Bone Level, diameter 3.3 mm, length 10 mm, at site 13; 1 × Bone Level, diameter 4.1 mm, length 10 mm, at sites 16 and 26; all Straumann, Basel, Switzerland). Implant axes and positions had been planned with the final screw-retained rehabilitation in mind. To speed up osseointegration, the selected implants featured a hydrophilic implant surface (Straumann SLActive®). Reduced-diameter implants are a commonly preferred choice after bone augmentation procedures to avoid excessive trauma during implant-bed preparation. After repositioning the flap and securing it with 5-0 nylon sutures, the implants were left to heal in a submerged position (Figs 17 to 22).

Fig 21   Submerged healing protocol.

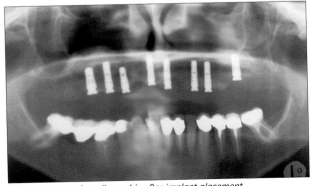

Fig 22   Panoramic radiographic after implant placement.

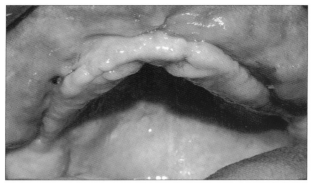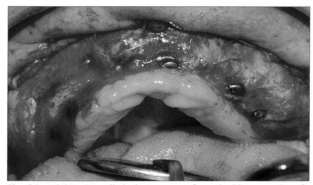

Fig 23   Clinical situation 3 months after implant surgery. Both the initial atrophy and the previous need for extensive periosteal releasing incisions had clearly resulted in loss of the buccal sulcus and a lack of keratinized mucosa.

Figs 24 and 25   A vestibuloplasty was performed with mucosal grafts taken from the palate, creating more favorable soft-tissue conditions in the peri-implant areas.

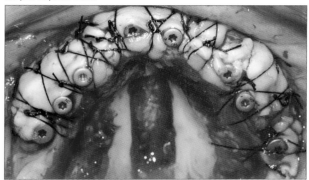

Fig 25

Postoperative instructions again included antibiotics for 1 week and chlorhexidine digluconate for 2 weeks.

Postoperative recovery was uneventful. The patient was not allowed to wear a removable prosthesis for 2 weeks. After that time, she was provided with a soft-relined denture.

Re-entry
The original plan had been to uncover the implants and commence the prosthetic phase 8 weeks after the implant procedure. Yet, as frequently observed in the wake of major reconstructions performed on severely resorbed bone, the buccal sulcus was reduced and the amount of keratinized buccal mucosa was inadequate (Fig 23).

Since the presence of a keratinized mucosal layer around implants is normally essential to soft-tissue stability and health, it was decided to perform a vestibuloplasty with free gingival grafts harvested from the palate. Grafts were placed labial to the implants and stabilized with crossed 5-0 silk sutures anchored to the periosteum. Osseointegration was confirmed for all implants. Cover screws were replaced by longer healing abutments, and the palatal donor sites were protected with a screw-retained resin device. This procedure was conducted under general anesthesia with nasotracheal intubation (Figs 24 and 25).

The sutures were removed after 2 weeks and the peri-implant soft tissues allowed to heal for another 2 weeks before initiating the prosthetic phase.

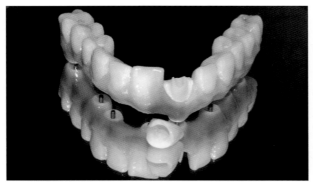 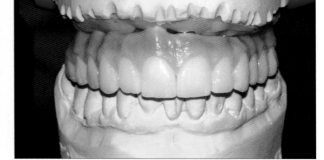

Figs 26 and 27   Final prosthesis prior to intraoral delivery.

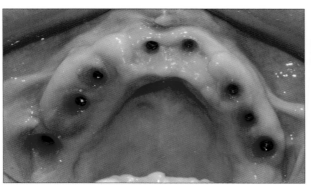 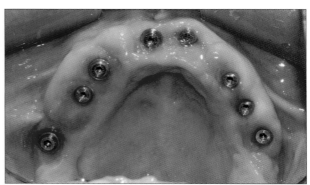

Figs 28 and 29   Intraoral occlusal view before and after connecting the abutments.

Prosthetic procedures

After taking impressions and interarch records, a screw-retained provisional prosthesis was fabricated to verify esthetics, perioral tissue support, function, and phonetics. Despite the bone reconstruction, it was necessary to incorporate a certain amount of artificial soft-tissue structure into this prosthetic design to combine the correct intermaxillary relationships with correct tooth dimensions. Photographs of the patient when she still had her teeth were used as a blueprint to restore the original tooth shapes.

Temporary abutments were used for the resin-based temporary prosthesis. Screw-retained superstructures are usually preferred for complex restorations, whether temporary or definitive. After delivery of the temporary fixed framework, the patient was instructed in oral hygiene procedures, including the use of dental floss. She wore this prosthesis for 6 months and provided very positive feedback about all aspects of the rehabilitation.

The same functional and esthetic parameters were used for the definitive rehabilitation.

Dental ceramics were layered onto a screw-retained zirconia framework implemented in CAD/CAM technology. The soft tissues were reproduced using pink porcelain (Figs 26 and 27). Multi-base abutments (NC and RC Multi-Base abutments; Straumann, Basel, Switzerland) were used as intermediate components connecting the definitive framework to the implants (Figs 28 and 29).

A cemented crown was selected for site 21 to avoid a suboptimal location of the screw access hole in this position. The access holes (Fig 30) were then sealed with a composite resin. Clinical views and a panoramic radiograph showing the final prosthesis in situ are provided in Figures 31 to 34.

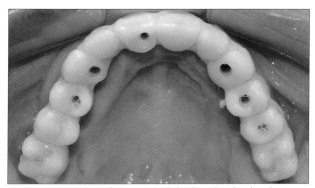

Fig 30   Occlusal view of the prosthesis in situ, also showing the access holes.

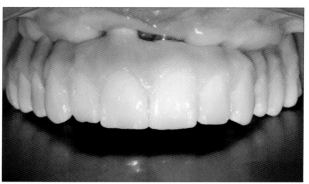

Fig 31   Close-up views of the final screw-retained prosthesis in situ.

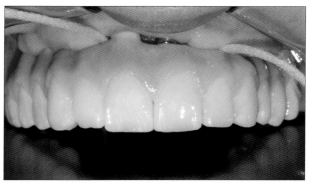

Fig 32   The patient was instructed to floss (Super-Floss, Oral-B) for inter-implant oral hygiene.

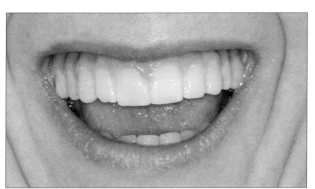

Fig 33   Portrait view of the patient's smile at the end of treatment.

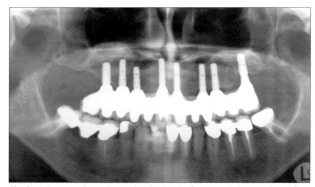

Fig 34   Panoramic radiograph obtained after the delivery of the final prosthesis.

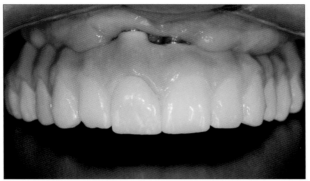

Figs 35 to 38   Clinical and radiographic situation 3 years after prosthetic delivery.

Follow-up

Follow-up and professional maintenance visits were scheduled at 6-month intervals. They confirmed an adequate level of plaque control and the absence of soft-tissue inflammation. The framework has been removed, cleaned, and disinfected once a year. Screw-retained rehabilitations are ideal from this viewpoint.

The 3-year clinical and radiographic follow-up confirmed an excellent functional and esthetic outcome. The grafted bone was stable and showed no signs of peri-implant resorption (Figs 35 to 38).

Acknowledgments

Laboratory procedures
Carlo Pedrinazzi, Roberto Colli – Milan, Italy

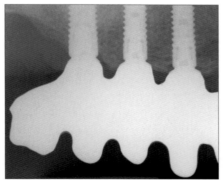

Fig 36

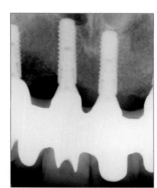

Fig 37

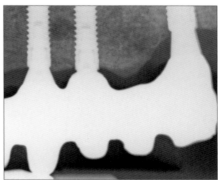

Fig 38

6.11 Iliac-Crest Block for Vertical and Horizontal Space Filling in the Anterior Maxilla

W. D. Polido, J. E. Roehe Neto

A 31-year-old man presented to our clinic 30 days after a motor vehicle accident in which he had suffered a dentoalveolar fracture in the anterior maxilla, including avulsion of teeth 12 and 11 and luxation of tooth 21. He was first treated on the night of the accident in a small city hospital with no oral and maxillofacial surgeon on the staff. A wired retention had been applied and the teeth repositioned to the best of the clinicians' abilities.

When he first presented to our care, the patient showed extrusion of teeth 12 and 11 associated with gingival recession due to bone loss in the anterior maxilla, and the stainless steel wires were still present (Figs 1 to 3).

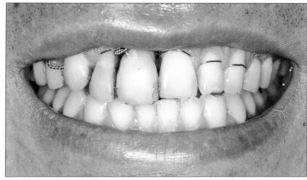

Fig 1   Initial clinical presentation, with wires to hold traumatized teeth in place. Smile-line view.

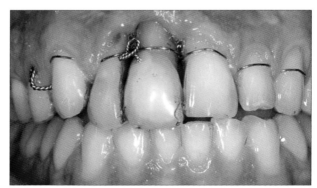

Fig 2   Buccal view.

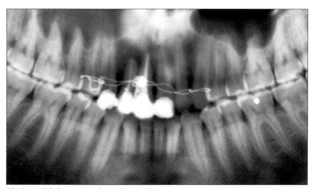

Fig 3   Initial panoramic radiograph.

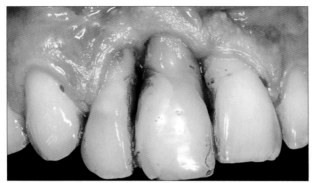

Fig 4   Anterior teeth after removal of containing wires.

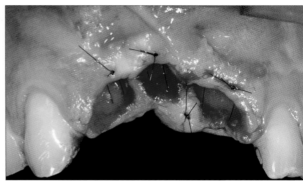

Fig 5   Clinical presentation after extraction treatment (anterior view).

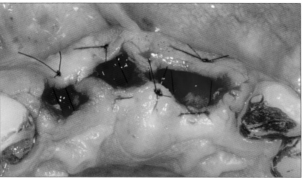

Fig 6   Occlusal view.

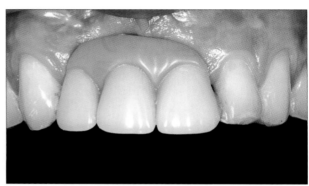

Fig 7   Removable partial denture (anterior view).

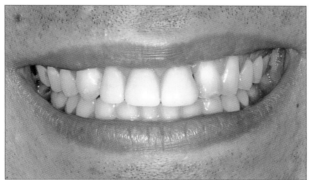

Fig 8   Removable partial denture (smile-line view).

The initial plan was to remove the affected teeth (12, 11, 21), provisionalization with a removable partial denture, and cleaning of the remaining teeth. This was performed in September 2004 (Figs 4 to 8).

After a healing period of 5 months, during which the patient quit smoking and was treated for other accident-related injuries (facial lacerations and ankle fracture), the plan for dental rehabilitation was initiated.

The preoperative clinical examination showed both vertical and horizontal osseous and soft-tissue defects (Figs 9 to 11). A new CT image was taken (Figs 12 and 13a-b) and three-dimensional planning performed with appropriate software available at the time (Dental Slice, Bioparts, DF, Brazil).

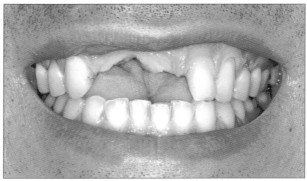
Fig 9   Smile-line view before bone grafting, 5 months after extraction.

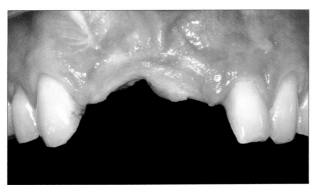
Fig 10   Buccal view.

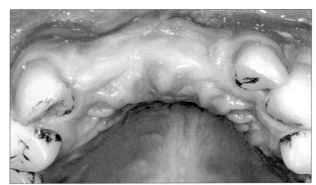
Fig 11   Occlusal view.

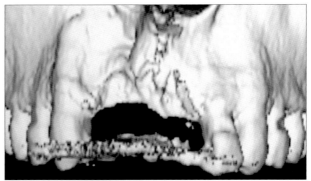
Fig 12   CT scan.

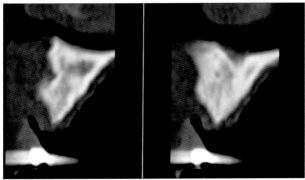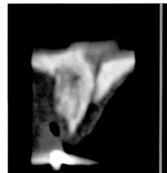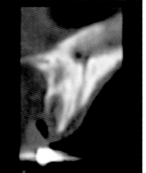
Figs 13a-b   Anterior cross-sectional views of the CT scan. Note the relationship with the radiopaque guide.

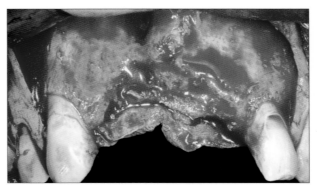

Fig 14   Intraoperative buccal view showing the osseous defect.

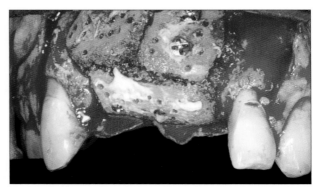

Fig 15   Corticocancellous bone grafts positioned and stabilized with screws. Anterior view.

Treatment plan

Three different plans were presented to the patient:

- Two implants at sites 12 and 21, with soft-tissue grafting and a dentogingival (i.e. including a pink component) three-unit fixed partial denture
- Distraction osteogenesis for vertical correction of the defect, and a second stage for a horizontal block graft from the ramus to correct the horizontal aspect. A soft-tissue graft was also considered.
- An autologous corticocancellous block graft from the iliac crest to simultaneously correct the vertical and horizontal deficiencies

The restoration originally envisioned in the second and third options consisted in a three-unit fixed partial denture on two implants.

After discussing risks and benefits of the three alternatives, keeping in mind the patient's young age and the perspective of the best possible restorative result, a decision was made in favor of the staged reconstruction with an iliac crest corticocancellous block graft.

Surgical reconstruction with block grafts

Surgery was performed under general anesthesia on an outpatient basis in March 2005. The iliac-crest graft was harvested from the left pelvis simultaneously with oral surgery.

A mucoperiosteal incision was performed from the distal of tooth 13 to the distal of tooth 22, followed by careful reflection and exposure of the defect (Fig 14). After removing all residual scar tissue, small perforations were performed at the host site with a size ¼ round bur to improve vascularization.

Three corticocancellous block grafts were carefully sculpted and adapted to the defect site. Two were positioned horizontally to reconstruct the natural curvature of the anterior maxilla, and one was positioned verti-

cally to gain bone height and allow for a restoration that would offer a natural appearance.

Before positioning the corticocancellous graft, a portion of cancellous graft chips was packed into the host area. Once the blocks were positioned with the cortical part facing the buccal and occlusal aspects, the grafts were fixated with a lag-screw (compressive) technique to squeeze the cancellous bone against the walls, thus eliminating any gaps between the block graft and the host site.

Before the grafts were secured, the cancellous part was slightly compressed to eliminate some of the fat content and reduce the lacunae. We consider these two steps very important and one of the main factors leading to graft success (excellent integration and less resorption).

With the grafts held in place with a clamp, two screws (diameter 2.0 mm; length 12 mm; Synthes, Davos, Switzerland) were positioned in each block using the lag-screw compressive technique (Figs 15 and 16). A perforation was performed with the 1.5-mm drill through the graft and recipient site and with the 1.8-mm drill through the graft only. Note that the screw must be long enough to engage the host site without perforating the palatal mucosa. After perforation, the screw size can be measured with a depth gauge.

The same principles were applied to fixate the vertical block. Care must be taken not to place the screw in the incisive canal. If possible, it is recommended to avoid placing the screws at the sites where the future implants will be positioned.

Once all blocks were fixated, the remaining cancellous bone was packed around them to fill any existing gaps.

Careful soft-tissue closure is of utmost importance. We performed a subperiosteal dissection as apically as possible, going laterally to the piriform aperture and almost

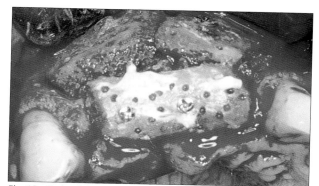

Figs 16   Occlusal view.

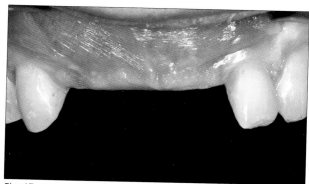

Figs 17   Anterior view 5 months after grafting, with complete healing of soft tissues and leveling of the defect.

as high as the infraorbital foramen. Dissecting subperiosteally rather than incising the periosteum can provide good soft-tissue release and maintain periosteal integrity. If necessary, small periosteal releasing incisions can be made, first extending superiorly the lateral releasing incisions, but only internally in the periosteum, without cutting the mucosa. Complete and passive adaptation of the soft tissue needs to be achieved, without excessive pull or periosteal incisions. This is another critical surgical step while frequently getting overlooked by surgeons who are worried only about the bone.

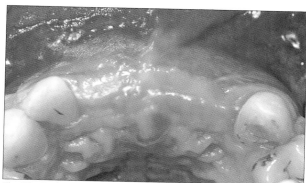

Figs 18   Occlusal view.

In this case, closing was performed with 4-0 mononylon sutures, which were removed 15 days after surgery. A 4-0 Vicryl suture may also be applied. The patient agreed to postpone wearing the removable partial denture for 7 days to avoid soft-tissue compression. After 7 days, the removable partial denture was adjusted to reduce its volume, and a soft relining material was added.

After 5 months of uneventful graft healing, a new CT image revealed complete adaptation of the graft and the volume of the three-dimensional reconstruction (Figs 17 to 19). Soft-tissue adaptation was also considered very good.

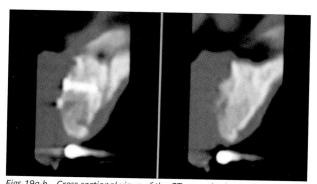

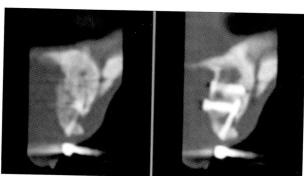

Figs 19a-b   Cross-sectional views of the CT scan obtained after grafting and before implant placement. Notice the relationship with the radiopaque and surgical guide. Compare with Figure 13.

Implant options

Implant and restorative options were again discussed with the patient. Two implants and a three-unit fixed partial denture were the first choice, but the possibility of three single units was also proposed.

Several factors were taken into account when considering the option of three single units: the success of the vertical and horizontal reconstruction, the smile line of the patient, the large mesiodistal span the form of the future teeth (more square than triangular), and the low distance from the contact point to the bone all spoke in favor of this choice. Potential lack of interimplant papillae was a major problem and was discussed in depth with the patient. However, the fact that he was young, had lost his teeth due to trauma rather than lack of care, had undergone a major reconstruction, and was willing to have individual teeth rather than a bridge, also were factors in the decision, as were the costs of the procedures.

After diagnostic waxing and construction of a surgical splint, the decision was made to place three implants for teeth 12, 11 and 21 in order to have single-unit restorations. This case was treated in 2005, when only the soft-tissue level Standard Plus (SP) implants by Straumann were available.

The choice was for two tapered-effect implants (Standard Plus TE SLActive®, diameter 3.3 mm, length 10 mm TE; Straumann, Basel, Switzerland) at sites 11 and 21, and one narrow-neck implant (Standard Plus NN SLActive®, diameter 3.3 mm, length 10 mm; Straumann, Basel, Switzerland) at site 12. Nowadays, our choice would have been for bone-level implants, possibly in the form of three Roxolid® Bone Level NC implants.

Implant surgery and healing

Implant surgery was performed under local anesthesia in September 2005, using a single stage to remove the fixation screws and to place the implants. During implant surgery, it was evident that the head of the fixation screw was flush with the bone, having retained almost exactly the same position as during the reconstructive procedure 5 months earlier (Figs 20 and 21). This was a clinical sign that little remodeling and resorption had taken place with the surgical technique used. Moreover, bone density was excellent, allowing for a single-stage technique and a 6-week period of osseointegration routinely used with SLA surfaces.

The implants were placed in the usual manner. The choice for the TE implant was to improve primary stability.

The mesiodistal space was appropriate to place three implants, and the patient agreed that a potential lack of interdental papillae was acceptable given the anatomy of his teeth and the single-unit rehabilitation strategy (Figs 22 to 24).

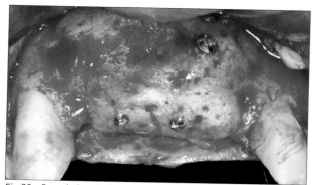

Fig 20   Buccal view during implant surgery. The screw heads are flush with the bone.

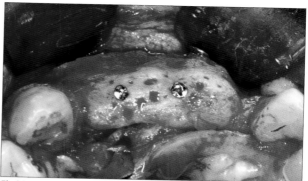

Fig 21   Occlusal view during implant surgery.

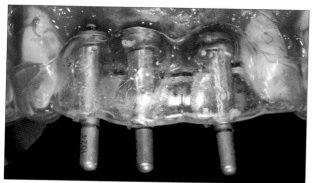

Figs 22a-b   Surgical guide with direction indicator pins.

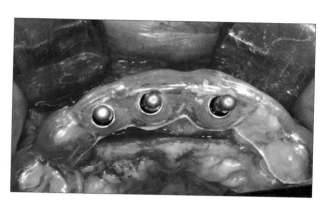

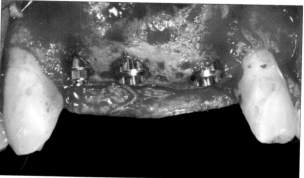

Fig 23   Buccal view during implant surgery.

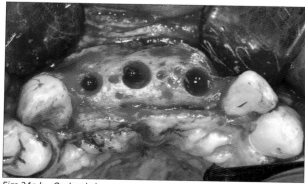

Figs 24a-b   Occlusal view.

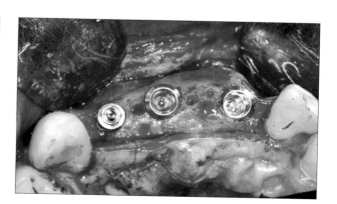

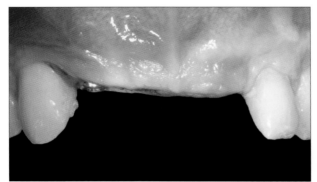

Fig 25   Buccal view 2 months after implant placement.

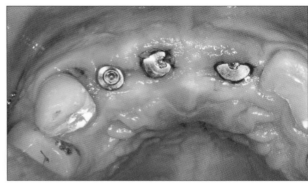

Fig 26   Occlusal view 2 months after implant placement.

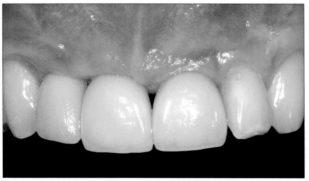

Figs 27a-b   Final restoration with single-tooth metal-ceramic crowns.

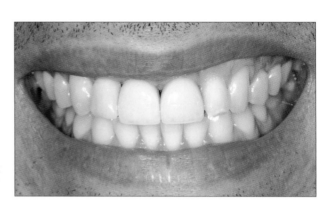

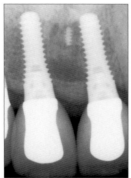 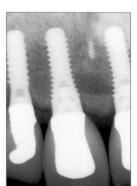

Figs 28a-b   Periapical radiographs taken at final restoration delivery.

After 8 weeks, healing was uneventful (Figs 25 and 26). Impressions were taken, with the ensuing restorative procedures (including provisionals) taking around 3 months.

In February 2006, three single-unit, screw-retained, metal-ceramic restorations were placed using SynOcta® abutments (Straumann, Basel, Switzerland) (Figs 27 and 28).

Follow-up

The patient returned for follow-up examinations after 18 months in August 2007 (Figs 29a-c and 30a-b), after 3.5 years in June 2009 (Figs 31a-c), and after 6 years in March 2012 (Figs 32a-c and 33a-b). Minor remodeling in the horizontal aspect was noticed after 6 years, but the vertical aspect was completely stable. Clinical pictures and periapical radiographs show stable results after 6 years of loading.

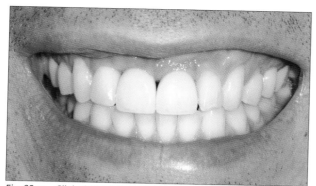

Figs 29a-c   Clinical view, 18-month follow-up in August 2007.

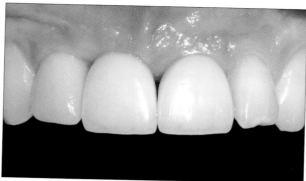

Fig 29b

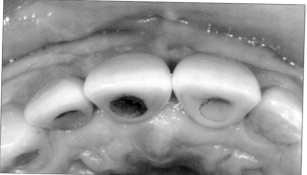

Fig 29c

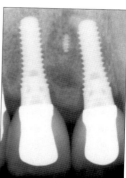

Figs 30a-b   Periapical radiographs, 18-month follow-up in August 2007.

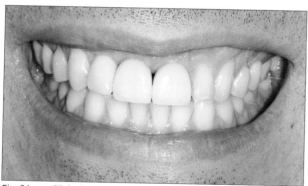

Figs 31a-c   Clinical view, 40-month follow-up in June 2009.

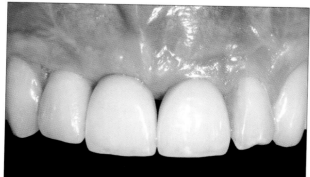

Fig 31b

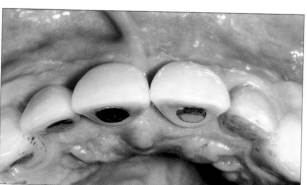

Fig 31c

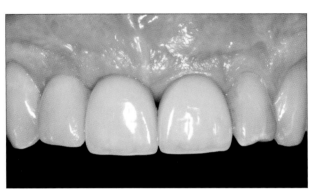

Figs 32a-c   Clinical view, 6-year follow-up in March 2012.

Acknowledgments

Orthopedic surgery (iliac-crest graft harvesting) procedures
Felipe Wildt do Canto, MD – Porto Alegre, RS, Brazil

Prosthodontic procedures
João Emilio Roehe Neto, DDS, Prosthetic Dentistry – Porto Alegre, RS, Brazil

Laboratory procedures
PROTEM - Dental laboratory – Porto Alegre, RS, Brazil

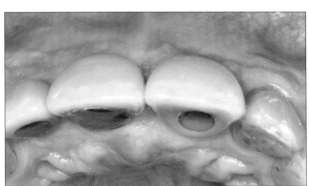

Fig 32b

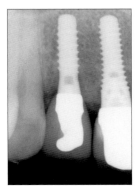

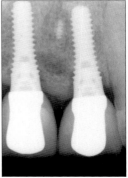

Figs 33a-b   Periapical radiographs, 6-year follow-up in March 2012.

Table 1   Esthetic Risk Assessment (ERA) of the initial presentation

Esthetic Risk Factors	Level of Risk		
	Low	Moderate	High
Medical status	Healthy, cooperative patient with an intact immune system		Reduced immune system
Smoking habit	Non-smoker	Light smoker (< 10 cig/day)	Heavy smoker (≥ 10 cig/day)
Patient's esthetic expectations	Low	Medium	High
Lip line	Low	Medium	High
Gingival biotype	Low-scalloped, thick	Medium-scalloped, medium thick	High-scalloped thin
Shape of tooth crowns	Rectangular		Triangular
Infection at implant site	None	Chronic	Acute
Bone level at adjacent teeth	≤ 5 mm to contact point	5.5 to 6.5 mm to contact point	≥ 7 mm to contact point
Restorative status of neighboring teeth	Virgin		Restored
Width of edentulous span	1 tooth (≥ 7 mm) 1 tooth (≥ 5.5 mm)	1 tooth (< 7 mm) 1 tooth (< 5.5 mm)	2 teeth or more
Soft-tissue anatomy	Intact soft tissue		Soft-tissue defects
Bone anatomy of alveolar crest	Alveolar crest without bone deficiency	Horizontal bone deficiency	Vertical bone deficiency

6.12 Le Fort I Interpositional Graft and Mandibular Sandwich Osteotomy for Maxillofacial Rehabilitation after Severe Periodontitis

H. Terheyden

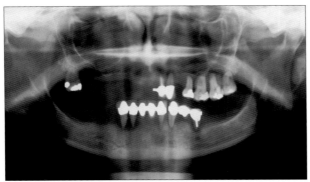

Fig 1 Panoramic radiograph showing a failing dentition after chronic periodontitis. Vertical bone loss was 6 to 8 mm.

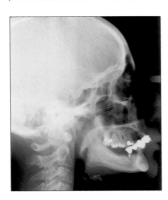

Fig 2 Lateral cephalogram showing that the vertical dimension of occlusion was dramatically reduced.

A 47-year-old woman who had suffered from aggressive periodontitis requiring a number of periodontal interventions over more than 10 years was referred by her general dental practitioner and periodontologist for bone augmentation and implant therapy. Her failing dentition had already been scheduled for extraction. The patient expressed a desire for implant-supported fixed restorations and esthetic improvement of her lower face. She had agreed to consult with a maxillofacial surgeon after the referring dentist had suggested bone augmentation.

An initial examination by the maxillofacial surgeon revealed mobility of all residual teeth in a patient who was very unhappy with the function of her removable partial dentures (Figs 1 and 2). Due to periodontally migrated flaring teeth and loss of occlusal support, the vertical dimension of occlusion was dramatically reduced. The patient was displeased with her lower face because of deepened nasolabial, commissural, and supramental folds. The radiographs indicated vertical bone loss of 6 mm in the mandible and 8 mm in the maxilla on average.

The patient's medical history did not reveal any severe systemic diseases or increased risks of surgical procedures conducted under general anesthesia. She did not smoke, had been under periodontal supervision for many years, and was well motivated to comply with oral hygiene requirements. Following previous consultations with her dentist, her expectations of surgery and attainable improvements were realistic. The patient was a small business owner and had realistic expectations about limitations related to workloads and chewing. She did express a desire to resume her leisure sports activities as soon as possible after bone harvesting. A detailed cost estimate was presented and agreed on.

After scheduling a team meeting with the referring dentist, it was agreed to proceed with the following treatment plan:

- Diagnostic wax-up with an increased vertical dimension of occlusion
- Fabrication of temporary complete dentures for the maxilla and mandible
- Extraction of all residual teeth
- Immediate provision of the temporary complete dentures
- Four months after extraction surgery: bone augmentation surgery with a bone substitute and a small amount of iliac bone to increase the vertical dimension of the mandibular crest by 6 mm and the vertical dimension of the maxillary crest by 8 mm
- Four months after augmentation surgery: removal of the osteosynthesis material, implant surgery
- Four months after implant surgery: uncovering of the implants soft-tissue surgery to improve the attached mucosal tissues
- Prosthetic treatment
- Recall

The patient gave her informed consent based on detailed information about typical risks and adverse effects of the surgical treatment, also including requirements for postoperative behavior, limitations to occupational activities, any treatment alternatives (including the option of no treatment), and the estimated cost of treatment. A second informed consent was obtained by the anesthesiologist who would perform the general anesthesia.

The extraction sockets were found to heal quickly within the 4-month period after tooth extraction. It was mandatory for the jawbone to be consolidated by the time of performing the segmental osteotomies. One should always wait, as spontaneous bone regeneration will often turn out more pronounced than expected from initial radiographs (Figs 3 and 4).

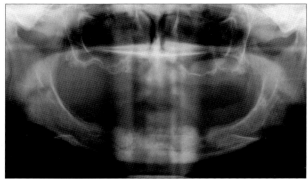

Fig 3   Panoramic radiograph obtained 4 months after extraction.

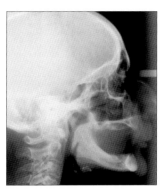

Fig 4   Lateral cephalogram obtained 4 months after extraction.

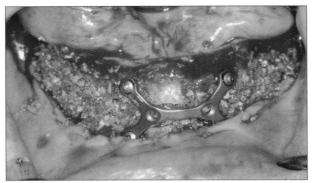

Fig 5 *Mandibular surgery after horizontal sandwich osteotomy, osteosynthesis, and filling of the gap with a mixture of Bio-Oss® and 25% iliac bone chips. A midline crestal incision in the linea alba had been was used.*

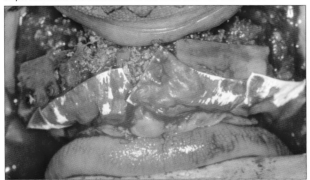

Fig 6 *Maxilla after bilateral preparation of the sinus membranes and Le Fort I osteotomy with downfracture and slight advancement. The Le Fort I interpositional gap was filled with a mixture of 75% Bio-Oss® and 25% iliac-bone chips. Two iliac-bone blocks were additionally placed to augment and reinforce the ridge at the canine sites (cornerstone principle). Bio-Gide® membranes bolstered the flaps.*

Augmentation surgery was performed on an inpatient basis, with the patient hospitalized for 5 days. A two-team approach was taken for iliac-bone harvesting and intraoral surgery, both with the patient under general anesthesia by nasal intubation. Using a short 3-cm incision, two monocortical blocks were harvested from the inner iliac table with an oscillating saw and around 10 cm³ of cancellous bone with a curette. Midcrestal incisions were used to simultaneously expose both jaws precisely in the linea alba by splitting the existing attached mucosa in two. In the mandible, the horizontal bone cut was made with an oscillating saw, carefully keeping the crestal and lingual tissues attached for blood perfusion of the segment, which was then raised by 6 mm and stabilized with an X-shaped 2.0-mm titanium miniplate (Martin, Tuttlingen, Germany). Additional 2-mm positioning screws were used to secure the segment in the posterior jaw. The interpositional gap was filled with a mixture of 75% bovine bone particles, 1–2 mm in size (Bio-Oss®; Geistlich Biomaterials, Wolhusen, Switzerland) and 25% ground cancellous bone from the iliac crest (Fig 5).

Then a resorbable collagen membrane (Bio-Gide®; Geistlich Biomaterials) was placed over the interpositional gap and underneath the suture line, using 40 polyamide pseudomonofil material (Supramid®; Resorba, Nürnberg, Germany). The procedure in the maxilla was started by performing conventional preparations of the sinus membranes through a lateral osteotomy using diamond burs. After elevating the sinus membrane and the nasal mucosa, the canine buttress of the maxilla was cut with a Lindemann bur. Masing chisels were used on the lateral nasal duct walls and septum chisels on the nasal septum, then detaching the maxilla with an Obwegeser chisel from the pterygoid processes for downfracture. After carefully dissecting and preserving both of the greater palatine arteries, the maxilla was carefully mobilized, slightly advanced, and stabilized to an elevated height of 8 mm with two L-shaped 2-mm titanium miniplates and 5-mm bone screws. The same grafting mixture as in the mandible was used to fill the interpositional gap and the sinus floors. A total of 10 g of bone substitute were used. An additional grafting measure taken only for the maxillary reconstruction was to place two iliac bone blocks at the canine sites, thus reinforcing the atrophic jaw in those areas and bridging the interpositional gap with solid bone (Fig 6).

Bio-Gide membranes were placed both over the grafts and underneath the sutures in the maxilla. Discharged from the hospital after four days postoperatively, the patient was able to move freely, using one crutch, without limitations to the load-bearing capacity of her limbs. After 6 weeks, she was able to move without any pain and could resume her leisure sports activities. She was allowed to use removable dentures but was asked not to chew with them and to remain on a soft diet. The vertical gains had remained stable (Figs 7 and 8).

Four months later, the osteosynthesis materials were removed under general anesthesia on an outpatient basis. In accordance with the initial setup, which had been transferred to a drill guide via the provisional denture, eight cylinder-type screws (lengths 11 to 13 mm; Camlog, Wimsheim, Germany) were placed in the maxilla and six in the mandible (Figs 9 and 10).

A minor need for re-grafting at site 46 was met with some bone from the chin area and a Bio-Gide membrane. The bone augmentation achieved was sufficient to ensure that parallel implant positions could be attained as envisioned in the drill guide, as parallelism between the resultant prosthetic tooth axes will facilitate the prosthetic and laboratory procedures.

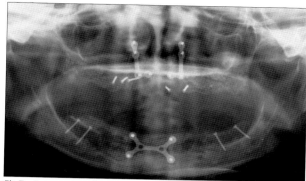

Fig 7   Panoramic radiograph after augmentation surgery.

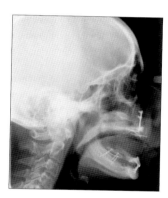

Fig 8   Lateral cephalogram after augmentation surgery.

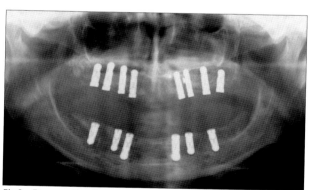

Fig 9   Four months after augmentation surgery, implants of considerable length were placed, taking advantage of the newly gained vertical bone dimensions.

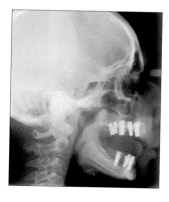

Fig 10   Lateral cephalogram after implant surgery.

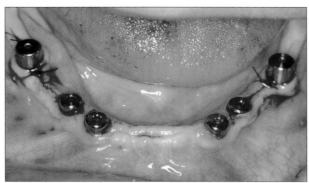

Fig 11   Lower implants after re-entry. Thanks to the conservative midcrestal incision, equal amounts of natural attached mucosa were available on both sides of the dental implants. There was no need for soft-tissue grafting or vestibuloplasty.

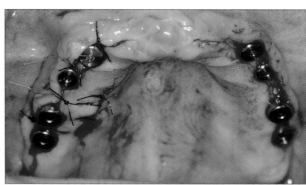

Fig 12   Thanks to the conservative midcrestal incision, sufficient amounts of natural attached mucosa were available on the buccal side of the dental implants. There was no need for soft-tissue grafting or vestibuloplasty.

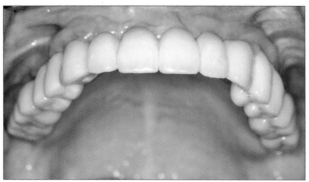

Fig 13   Fixed prosthesis (zirconia base) in the maxilla.

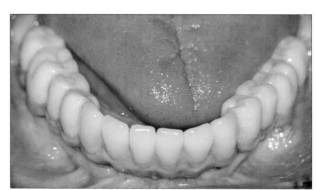

Fig 14   Removable prosthesis (zirconia base) in the mandible.

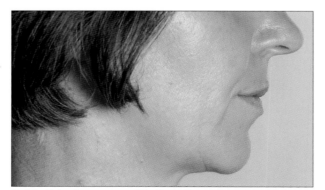

Fig 15   Natural appearance of the lip profile and lower facial third.

After a waiting period of 4 months, the implants were uncovered. Once again, the same midcrestal incisions were used. Since these had been designed from the outset to match the implants, every implant was now surrounded by attached mucosa (Figs 11 and 12). Site 13 was found to be associated with thin mucosa and, therefore, was additionally treated with a subepithelial connective-tissue graft 1 × 1 cm in size for reinforcement.

After 4 more weeks, prosthodontic treatment was initiated in the referring practitioner's office (Dr. Beata Simon, Hamburg, Germany). Zirconia-based fixed prostheses were delivered in both jaws (Figs 13 and 14).

The originally achieved gain in vertical dimension was deemed inadequate during try-ins. The patient's request for a greater vertical increase led to a design of her mandibular restoration that incorporated artificial gingiva. Delivery of the final restorations was found to restore the patient's lower face to a natural and juvenile appearance (Fig 15).

After scheduling a recall program, the patient has been followed up for 8 years at the time of writing this report (Figs 16 and 17). The prostheses continue to be fully functional without giving the patient discomfort or requiring repairs. There have been no adverse periodontal findings other than some bleeding on probing related to the implant at site 27 during the latest visit. The site responded well to local cleaning and disinfection.

Discussion

One way of compensating for periodontitis-induced loss of the vertical bone dimension is by prosthetic means, including options such as long crowns with artificial gingiva, saddle-style prostheses, or removable overdentures. The other strategy, as adopted in the case here presented, is to replace the lost tissue structures by surgical means.

Vertical bone augmentation had several advantages in this patient, one example being the natural appearance of short anterior maxillary crowns emerging from a natural attached mucosa. Rather than using removable dentures, it was both technically simpler and allowed for all-ceramic restorations to implement the superstructures as fixed prostheses. All this made it much easier for the patient to accept the surgical and financial implications of bone augmentation treatment.

Interpositional grafting is an interesting alternative to traditional techniques of vertical bone augmentation like onlay grafting or guided bone regeneration (GBR). The concept is not new—with early reports on the use of "sandwich osteoplasty" in the maxilla and mandible dating back to Bell and coworkers (1977) and Schettler (1976)—and has been shown to yield excellent long-term results (Nyström and coworkers 2009; Chiapasco and coworkers 2009). What is new about the case here presented is that the Le Fort I osteotomy was combined with sinus floor elevation. Preserving the intact sinus membrane created a contained space secluded from the sinus and nasal cavity that could be filled with particulate materials.

Another new aspect about this case is the use of a bone substitute to fill the interpositional space. From a biological viewpoint, onlay grafting or GBR only involves unilateral contact between the graft and vital bone, whereas the contact of an interpositional graft with perfused bone marrow is bilateral, which facilitates and expedites integration of the graft with new bone via blood vessels and bone cells. The fact that the interpositional situation with a gap configuration like the one observed in the present case can eliminate the need for iliacblock grafts will increase patient acceptance and reduce surgical donor-site trauma.

It is a major clinical benefit of the interpositional technique that the soft tissues remain attached to the oral

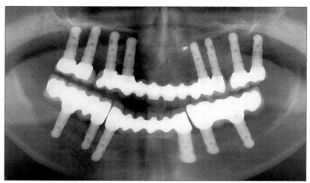

Fig 16 Panoramic radiograph at the 1-year follow-up. Stable peri-implant bone levels and no loss of vertically augmented bone volume.

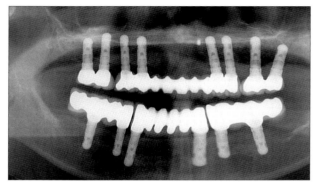

Fig 17 Panoramic radiograph at the 8-year follow-up. Continued stable peri-implant bone levels and no loss of vertically augmented bone volume.

aspect of the bone segment. As a result, the attached mucosa remains on top of the crest where it is needed for the emergence of the implant, reducing the need for additional softtissue surgery in comparison with onlay grafts.

Vertical onlay grafts on the edentulous ridges are prone to undergoing height resorption, with occasionally unpredictable consequences, over time (Chiapasco and coworkers 2009). The fact that bone grafts are better protected in interpositional than onlay situations adds to their stability. Also, no need to detach the soft tissues from the covering bone segment, at least not on the oral side, will reduce surface resorption. Accordingly, stable bone levels continue to be seen in the case here discussed even 8 years after interpositional grafting.

Acknowledgments

Prosthodontic procedures on recall
Beata Simon, Dr med dent – Hamburg, Germany

7 Management of Complications

H. Terheyden

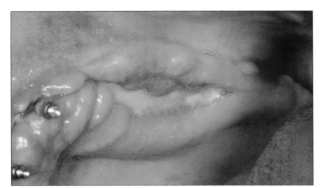

Fig 1a Wound dehiscence with exposure of an iliac onlay graft 2 weeks after augmentation. The patient did not report any tissue pain.

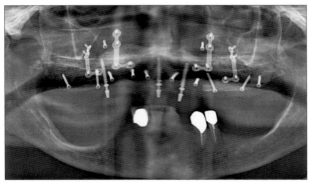

Fig 1b LeFort I interpositional grafting combined with iliac onlay grafts.

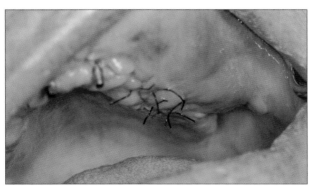

Fig 1c Clinical situation after salvage surgery and re-suturing of the flaps.

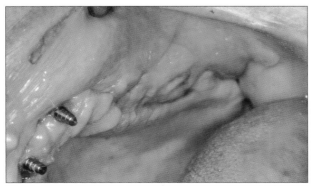

Fig 1d Further healing was uneventful. No recurrent wound dehiscence was noted.

Bone augmentation procedures are usually considered "advanced" or "complex" by the standards of the SAC classification. Any extensive surgery in atrophic ridges will place high demands on the skills not only of the surgeon but of the entire clinical team. A structured and well-organized clinical process is needed to perform complex procedures of this type, and the patient needs to understand and heed the recommendations given by the team.

Any of these complex surgical procedures must be preceded by proper case assessment, including a detailed study of the patient's medical history and adequate diagnostics. The first step of risk management must consist of evaluating the patient's general health, possibly in consultation with a physician, followed by appropriate surgical planning in consultation with the entire clinical team.

Patients cannot give their informed consent before being supplied with the necessary information, including typical risks and the nature of the more commonly observed potential complications, routine sequelae (inability to work, dietary restrictions, and the requirements of postoperative behavior), and cost estimates.

Implant surgery is elective surgery. Hence, the procedure should be scheduled to take place in an adequate environment at an ideal time. Appropriate materials and instrumentation must be used and the procedure carried out under sterile conditions. The patient should be provided with a list of medications and recommendations for postoperative behavior, none of which should leave any room for misunderstandings. There is also a need to draw up an organized aftercare plan with due precautions for emergency management.

Soft-tissue dehiscences

Soft-tissue dehiscences over grafts are a relatively frequent complication associated with augmentation surgery (Figs 1a,b). They are potentially hazardous in that they expose grafts and hardware to contaminants from the oral environment that may set the stage for graft loss.

Sutures tearing out of flap margins do not necessarily indicate an established wound infection. The collagen of the connective tissue in the wound margins undergoes continuous turnover by enzymatic degradation and fibroblast-induced new synthesis. This balance may shift through the action of proteolytic enzymes from neutrophils in connection with the physiologic inflammatory response that unfolds during early wound healing. Obviously, heavy bacterial inoculation of the wound is capable of boosting the neutrophilic reaction. Flap necrosis may be caused by factors interfering with arterial perfusion; examples are flap tension, overly tight sutures, or punctiform pressure (e.g. from sharp edges of a bone block).

The surgeon's response to any findings of flap dehiscence or necrosis should be to rinse the wound with a non-toxic antiseptic like polyvidone iodine and to consider systemic antibiotic therapy. The soft-tissue flaps can again be mobilized and re-sutured over the graft if palpation does not cause pain and the wound shows no putrid secretion, indicating that no manifest infection has developed. This maneuver is often successful and may salvage the graft (Figs 1a-d). Manifest infection should be treated by drainage and local disinfection therapy. The graft may need to be removed in cases of intractable infection, while healing by secondary intention may at least partially salvage an exposed graft.

Iliac-crest harvesting

Any harvesting of autologous grafts may be associated with donor site-related complications both intraoperatively and postoperatively. Potential intraoperative complications of iliac-crest procedures include fracture, perforation of the abdominal cavity, or blood loss, another typical complication being injuries to the genitofemoral nerve. Postoperative complications have been known to include gait disturbances, pain, and sensory disturbances in the lateral thigh area. Late fractures of the iliac wing should be suspected and excluded by radiograph on persistent gait pain lasting more than 4 weeks.

Intraoral bone harvesting

Both injuries to vessels or nerves and fractures, while being extremely rare, are nevertheless typical intraoperative risks of intraoral bone harvesting and augmentative surgery. Potential injuries to neighboring structures may affect teeth and the infraorbital, alveolar, or lingual nerves. Sensation and vitality loss in the anterior dentition has been reported to occur in 19% of procedures for chin-bone harvesting (Cordaro and coworkers 2011a).

In addition, late pathological mandibular fractures may occur even weeks after lateral bone harvesting after minor trauma has been inflicted. Great care should be exercised during the planning of osteotomies especially in osteoporotic patients, and suitable postoperative behavior will be required on the patient's part. Any deeper surgery performed in the maxilla should be expected to result in nosebleeds, which occasionally may be severe.

Severe complications

Complications both extremely rare and extremely severe would include intracerebral and intraorbital penetrations, blindness after maxillary surgery, and systemic or intracerebral infections. Also noteworthy is airway patency with respiratory insufficiency as a potential sequel to bleeding into the floor of the mouth or allergic swelling in the tongue or throat areas. Lastly, all surgical procedures related to dental implant treatment have in common the possibility of ingestion or aspiration of instruments or materials.

8   <u>Conclusions</u>

L. Cordaro, H. Terheyden

This book is part of the Treatment Guide series, introduced by the ITI to supply practitioners with the information they need in specific clinical situations in order to design and implement regimens of restorative treatment that involve the use of implants.

The authors of this volume have endeavored to offer comprehensive and evidence-based information on procedures of alveolar ridge augmentation in preparation for implant surgery. As discussed in Chapter 2, a large number of studies can be found in the literature that report on outcomes of augmentation techniques, but few of those authors reported on the initial defect characteristics to their readers. Based on the current body of information, it is almost impossible to derive a decision tree or an algorithm to guide practitioners in deciding on specific surgical approaches in specific clinical situations.

Most of the surgical techniques used to reconstruct deficient structures of alveolar bone in preparation for implants have been extensively discussed over the course of this book. Care has been taken to outline the rationale and indications for alveolar bone augmentation.

A variety of clinical case reports have been selected by the editors to illustrate the treatment philosophy that the ITI advocates in this field of implant dentistry. The procedures shown in these case reports have been performed by ITI fellows around the world. Although some cases with edentulous atrophic jaws have been included, most of the presentations deal with partially edentulous situations to reflect today's clinical reality in the dental office.

Treatment concepts have been clearly outlined. Staged procedures of reconstruction should be used whenever bone needs to be augmented outside of the bony envelope, while simultaneous procedures may be considered whenever soft-tissue support from adjacent bony structures is present and a major space-preserving effect is not required during healing of the graft. Some techniques such as bone splitting/expansion or distraction osteogenesis, while they have been mentioned, are so complex and technique-sensitive that they should be conducted exclusively by surgical teams that have considerable expertise in performing them.

Indications for techniques of intraoral and extraoral bone harvesting and the limitations of these approaches have been pointed out and discussed.

Large defects in alveolar bone remain a major challenge for dental implant surgeons around the world. While implant dentistry offers evidence-based solutions for a number of clinical situations, advanced or complex cases associated with severe bone loss will require the surgeon's judgment in selecting from a variety of surgical options and different materials.

The ITI has made an effort in this volume of the Treatment Guide series to offer an approach to alveolar-bone reconstructive surgery that is as systematic and reliable as can possibly be expected. The information provided, which has covered surgical solutions for all types of bone deficiencies, should make it possible for general dental practitioners to discuss with their patients any available options of bone reconstruction.

9 <u>References</u>

References have been listed in the order of (1) the first or only author's last name and (2) the year of publication. Identical short references are distinguished in the text by lowercase letters, which if used are listed in parentheses at the end of the respective entry.

Acocella A, Bertolai R, Colafranceschi M, Sacco R. Clinical, histological and histomorphometric evaluation of the healing of mandibular ramus bone block grafts for alveolar ridge augmentation before implant placement. J Craniomaxillofac Surg. **2010** Apr; 38(3): 222–230.

Adell R, Lekholm U, Gröndahl K, Brånemark PI, Lindström J, Jacobsson M. Reconstruction of severely resorbed edentulous maxillae using osseointegrated fixtures in immediate autogenous bone grafts. Int J Oral Maxillofac Implants. **1990** Fall; 5(3): 233–246.

Aghaloo TL, Moy PK. Which hard tissue augmentation techniques are the most successful in furnishing bony support for implant placement? Int J Oral Maxillofac Implants. **2007**; 22 Suppl: 49–70.

Al-Nawas B, Brägger U, Meijer HJ, Naert I, Persson R, Perucchi A, Quirynen M, Raghoebar GM, Reichert TE, Romeo E, Santing HJ, Schimmel M, Storelli S, ten Bruggenkate C, Vandekerckhove B, Wagner W, Wismeijer D, Müller F. A double-blind randomized controlled trial (RCT) of titanium-13 zirconium versus titanium grade IV small-diameter bone level implants in edentulous mandibles—results from a 1-year observation period. Clin Implant Dent Relat Res. **2012** Dec; 14(6): 896–904.

Anderson JM, Rodriguez A, Chang DT: Foreign body reaction to biomaterials. Semin Immunol. **2008** Apr; 20(2): 86–100.

Anitua E, Begoña L, Orive G. Clinical Evaluation of Split-Crest Technique with Ultrasonic Bone Surgery for Narrow Ridge Expansion: Status of Soft and Hard Tissues and Implant Success. Clin Implant Dent Relat Res. **2011** (Apr); 15(2): 176–187.

Annibali S, Cristalli MP, Dell'Aquila D, Bignozzi I, La Monaca G, Pilloni A. Short dental implants: a systematic review. J Dent Res. **2012** Jan; 91(1): 25–32.

Antoun H, Sitbon JM, Martinez H, Missika P. A prospective randomized study comparing two techniques of bone augmentation: onlay graft alone or associated with a membrane. Clin Oral Implants Res. **2001** Dec; 12(6): 632–639.

Araújo MG, Lindhe J.: Dimensional ridge alterations following tooth extraction. An experimental study in the dog. J Clin Periodontol. **2005** Feb; 32(2): 212–218.

Atieh MA, Zadeh H, Stanford CM, Cooper LF. Survival of short dental implants for treatment of posterior partial edentulism: a systematic review. Int J Oral Maxillofac Implants. **2012** Nov–Dec; 27(6): 1323–1331.

Augthun M, Yildirim M, Spiekermann H, Biesterfeld S. Healing of bone defects in combination with immediate implants using the membrane technique. Int J Oral Maxillofac Implants **1995** Jul–Aug; 10(3): 421–428.

Axhausen G. Histologische Untersuchungen über Knochentransplantationen am Menschen. [Histological studies of bone grafts in humans.] Deutsche Zeitschrift für Chirurgie. **1908** Dec; 91(3–4): 388–428.

Bahat O, Fontanessi RV. Efficacy of implant placement after bone grafting for three-dimensional reconstruction of the posterior jaw. Int J Periodontics Restorative Dent. **2001** Jun; 21(3): 220–231.

Barone A, Santini S, Sbordone L, Crespi R, Covani U. A clinical study of the outcomes and complications associated with maxillary sinus augmentation. Int J Oral Maxillofac Implants. **2006** Jan–Feb; 21(1): 81–85.

Barone A, Ricci M, Mangano F, Covani U. Morbidity associated with iliac crest harvesting in the treatment of maxillary and mandibular atrophies: a 10-year analysis. J Oral Maxillofac Surg. **2011** Sep; 69(9): 2298–2304.

Barter S, Stone P, Brägger U. A pilot study to evaluate the success and survival rate of titanium-zirconium implants in partially edentulous patients: results after 24 months of follow-up. Clin Oral Implants Res. **2012** Jul; 23(7): 873–881.

Becker J, Al-Nawas B, Klein MO, Schliephake H, Terheyden H, Schwarz F. Use of a new cross-linked collagen membrane for the treatment of dehiscence-type defects at titanium implants: a prospective, randomized-controlled double-blinded clinical multicenter study. Clin Oral Implants Res. **2009** Jul; 20(7): 742–749.

Bell WH, Buche WA, Kennedy JW 3rd, Ampil JP. Surgical correction of the atrophic alveolar ridge. A preliminary report on a new concept of treatment. Oral Surg Oral Med Oral Pathol. **1977** Apr; 43(4): 485 – 498.

Blanco J, Alonso A, Sanz M. Long-term results and survival rate of implants treated with guided bone regeneration: a 5-year case series prospective study. Clin Oral Implants Res. **2005** Jun; 16(3): 294 – 301.

Blus C, Szmukler-Moncler S. Split-crest and immediate implant placement with ultra-sonic bone surgery: a 3-year life-table analysis with 230 treated sites. Clin Oral Implants Res. **2006** Dec; 17(6): 700 – 707.

Bonewald LF. The amazing osteocyte. J Bone Miner Res. **2011** Feb; 26(2): 229 – 238.

Bornstein M, Cionca N, Mombelli A. Systemic Conditions and Treatments as Risks for Implant Therapy. Int J Oral Maxillofac Implants. **2009**; 24 (Suppl): 12 – 27.

Bosshardt D, Hjørting-Hansen E, Buser D. The fate of the autogenous bone graft. Forum Implantologicum. **2009**; 5(1): 4 – 11.

Bosshard D, Schenk R. Biologic basis of bone regeneration. In: Buser D (ed.). 20 years of guided bone regeneration in implant dentistry, 2nd ed. Chicago: Quintessence; **2010**.

Braut V, Bornstein MM, Lauber R, Buser D. Bone dimensions in the posterior mandible – a retrospective radiographic study using cone beam computed tomography. Part A: Analysis of the dentate sites. Int J Periodont Restorative Dent. **2012** Apr; 32(2): 175 – 184.

Burchardt H, Enneking WF. Transplantation of bone. Surg Clin North Am. **1978** Apr; 58 (2): 403 – 427.

Burchardt H. The biology of bone graft repair. Clin Orthop Relat Res. **1983** Apr; (174): 28 – 42.

Buser D, Brägger U, Lang NP, Nyman S. Regeneration and enlargement of jaw bone using guided tissue regeneration. Clin Oral Implants Res **1990** Dec; 1(1): 22 – 32.

Buser D, Dula K, Belser U, Hirt HP, Berthold H. Localized ridge augmentation using guided bone regeneration. I. Surgical procedure in the maxilla. Int J Periodontics Restorative Dent **1993**; 13(1): 29 – 45.

Buser D, Dula K, Belser UC, Hirt HP, Berthold H. Localized ridge augmentation using guided bone regeneration. II. Surgical procedure in the mandible. Int J Periodont Rest Dent. **1995** Feb; 15(1): 13 – 29.

Buser D, Dula K, Hirt HP, Schenk RK. Lateral ridge augmentation using autografts and barrier membranes: a clinical study with 40 partially edentulous patients. J Oral Maxillofac Surg. **1996** Apr; 54(4): 420 – 432; discussion 432 – 433.

Buser D, Mericske-Stern R, Bernard JP, Behneke A, Behneke N, Hirt HP, Belser UC, Lang NP. Long-term evaluation of non-submerged ITI implants. Part 1: 8-year life table analysis of a prospective multi-center study with 2359 implants. Clin Oral Implants Res. **1997** Jun; 8(3): 161 – 172.

Buser D, Ingimarsson S, Dula K, Lussi A, Hirt HP, Belser UC. Long-term stability of osseointegrated implants in augmented bone: a 5-year prospective study in partially edentulous patients. Int J Periodontics Restorative Dent. **2002** Apr; 22(4): 109 – 117.

Buser D, Martin W, Belser UC. Optimizing esthetics for implant restorations in the anterior maxilla: Anatomic and surgical considerations. Int J Oral Maxillofac Implants. **2004**; 19(suppl): 43 – 61.

Buser D, Chen ST, Weber HP, Belser UC. The concept of early implant placement following single tooth extraction in the esthetic zone: Biologic rationale and surgical procedures. Int J Periodont Rest Dent. **2008** Oct; 28(5): 440 – 451.

Buser D. Implant placement with simultaneous guided bone regeneration: Selection of biomaterials and surgical principles. In: Buser D (ed): 20 years of guided bone regeneration in implant dentistry. 2nd ed. Chicago: Quintessence; **2009**: 123 – 152.

Çakur B, Dağistan S, Miloğlu Ö, Bilge M. Nonsyndromic oligodontia in permanent dentition: three siblings. The Internet Journal of Dental Science. **2006**; 3(2). Retrieved 1 Nov 2011.

Carpio L, Loza J, Lynch S, Genco R. Guided bone regeneration around endosseous implants with anorganic bovine bone mineral. A randomized controlled trial comparing bioabsorbable versus non-resorbable barriers. J Periodontol. **2000** Nov; 71(11): 1743 – 1749.

Casentini P, Wismeijer D, Chiapasco M: Treatment options for the edentulous arch. In: Wismeijer D, Casentini P, Gallucci G, Chiapasco M (eds). Loading protocols in implant dentistry – edentulous patients. ITI Treatment Guide, Vol 4 Berlin: Quintessence; **2010**: 45 – 56.

Castagna L, Polido WD, Soares LG, Tinoco EM. Tomographic evaluation of iliac crest bone grafting and the use of immediate temporary implants to the atrophic maxilla. Int Oral Maxillofac Surg. **2013** Sep; 42(9): 1067 – 1072.

Cawood JI, Howell RA. A classification of the edentulous jaws. Int J Oral Maxillofac Surg. **1988** Aug; 17(4): 232 – 236.

Chaushu G, Blinder D, Taicher S, Chaushu S. The effect of precise reattachment of the mentalis muscle on the soft tissue response to genioplasty. J Oral Maxillofac Surg. **2001** May; 59(5): 510 – 516; discussion 517.

Chen S, Buser D. Recommendations for selecting the treatment approach. In: Buser D, Wismeijer D, Belser UC (eds): Implant placement in post-extraction sites: Treatment options. ITI Treatment Guide, Vol 3. Berlin: Quintessence; **2008**: 38 – 42, 2008.

Chen ST, Buser D. Clinical and esthetic outcomes of implants placed in postextraction sites. Int J Oral Maxillofac Implants **2009**; 24 Suppl: 186 – 217.

Chiapasco M, Abati S, Romeo E, Vogel G. Clinical outcome of autogenous bone blocks or guided bone regeneration with e-PTFE membranes for the reconstruction of narrow edentulous ridges. Clin Oral Implants Res. **1999** Aug; 10(4): 278 – 288.

Chiapasco M, Consolo U, Bianchi A, Ronchi P. Alveolar distraction osteogenesis for the correction of vertically deficient edentulous ridges: a multicenter prospective study on humans. Int J Oral Maxillofac Implants. **2004** May – Jun; 19(3): 399 – 407.

Chiapasco M, Ferrini F, Casentini P, Accardi S, Zaniboni M. Dental implants placed in expanded narrow edentulous ridges with the Extension Crest device. A 1 – 3-year multicenter follow-up study. Clin Oral Implants Res. **2006** Jun; 17(3): 265 – 272. (a)

Chiapasco M, Zaniboni M, Boisco M. Augmentation procedures for the rehabilitation of deficient edentulous ridges with oral implants. Clin Oral Implants Res. **2006** Oct; 17 Suppl 2: 136 – 159. (b)

Chiapasco M, Brusati R, Ronchi P. Le Fort I osteotomy with interpositional bone grafts and delayed dental implants for the rehabilitation of extremely atrophied maxillae: a 1 – 9-year clinical follow-up study on humans. Clin Oral Implants Res. **2007** Feb; 18(1): 74 – 85. (a)

Chiapasco M, Zaniboni M, Rimondini L. Autogenous onlay bone grafts vs. alveolar distraction osteogenesis for the correction of vertically deficient edentulous ridges: a 2 – 4-year prospective study on humans. Clin Oral Implants Res. **2007** Aug; 18(4): 432 – 440. (b)

Chiapasco M, Casentini P, Zaniboni M. Bone augmentation procedures in implant dentistry. Int J Oral Maxillofac Implants. **2009**; 24 Suppl: 237 – 259.

Chiapasco M, Casentini P, Zaniboni M, Corsi E. Evaluation of peri-implant bone resorption around Straumann Bone Level implants placed in areas reconstructed with autogenous vertical onlay bone grafts. Clin Oral Implants Res. **2012** Sep; 23(9): 1012 – 1021. (a)

Chiapasco M, Casentini P, Zaniboni M, Corsi E, Anello T. Titanium-zirconium alloy narrow-diameter implants (Straumann Roxolid®) for the rehabilitation of horizontally deficient edentulous ridges: prospective study on 18 consecutive patients. Clin Oral Implants Res. **2012** Oct; 23(10): 1136 – 1141. (b)

Chiapasco M, Autelitano L, Rabbiosi D, Zaniboni M. The role of pericranium grafts in the reduction of postoperative dehiscences and bone resorption after reconstruction of severely deficient edentulous ridges with autogenous onlay bone grafts. Clin Oral Implants Res. **2013** Jun; 24(6): 679 – 687.

Clavero J, Lundgren S. Ramus or chin grafts for maxillary sinus inlay and local onlay augmentation: Comparison of donor site morbidity and complications. Clin Implant Dent Relat Res. **2003**; 5: 154 – 160.

Colella G, Cannavale R, Pentenero M, Gandolfo S. Oral implants in radiated patients: a systematic review. Int J Oral Maxillofac Implants. **2007** Jul – Aug; 22(4): 616 – 622.

Cordaro L, Amadé DS, Cordaro M. Clinical results of alveolar ridge augmentation with mandibular block bone grafts in partially edentulous patients prior to implant placement. Clin Oral Implants Res. **2002**; 13: 103 – 111.

Cordaro L. Bilateral simultaneous augmentation of the maxillary sinus floor with particulated mandible. Report of a technique and preliminary results. Clin Oral Implants Res. **2003** Apr; 14(2): 201 – 206.

Cordaro L, Torsello F, Accorsi Ribeiro C, Liberatore M, Mirisola di Torresanto V. Inlay-onlay grafting for three-dimensional reconstruction of the posterior atrophic maxilla with mandibular bone. Int J Oral Maxillofac Surg. **2010** Apr; 39(4): 350 – 357.

Cordaro L, Torsello F, Miuccio MT, di Torresanto VM, El-iopoulos D. Mandibular bone harvesting for alveolar reconstruction and implant placement: subjective and objective cross-sectional evaluation of donor and recipient site up to 4 years. Clin Oral Implants Res. **2011** Nov; 22(11): 1320 – 1326. (a)

Cordaro L, Torsello F, Morcavallo S, di Torresanto VM. Effect of bovine bone and collagen membranes on healing of mandibular bone blocks: a prospective randomized controlled study. Clin Oral Implants Res. **2011** Oct; 22(1): 1145 – 1150. (b)

Cordaro L, Boghi F, Mirisola di Torresanto V, Torsello F. Reconstruction of the moderately atrophic edentulous maxilla with mandibular bone grafts. Clin Oral Impl Res. **2012** Jul 13. [Epub ahead of print] (a)

Cordaro L, Torsello F, Chen S, Ganeles J, Brägger U, Hämmerle C. Implant-supported single tooth restoration in the aesthetic zone: transmucosal and submerged healing provide similar outcome when simultaneous bone augmentation is needed. Clin Oral Implants Res. **2012** Jun 15. [Epub ahead of print] (b)

Dahlin C, Sennerby L, Lekholm U, Linde A, Nyman S. Generation of new bone around titanium implants using a membrane technique: An experimental study in rabbits. Int J Oral Maxillofac Implants. **1988** Spring; 4(1): 19 – 25.

Dahlin C, Sennerby L, Lekholm U, Linde A, Nyman S. Generation of new bone around titanium implants using a membrane technique: an experimental study in rabbits. Int J Oral Maxillofac Implants. **1989** Spring; 4(1): 19 – 25.

Dahlin C, Gottlow J, Linde A, Nyman S. Healing of maxillary and mandibular bone defects using a membrane technique. An experimental study in monkeys. Scand J Plast Reconstr Surg Hand Surg. **1990**; 24(1): 13 – 19.

Dahlin C, Lekholm U, Becker W, Becker B, Higuchi K, Callens A, van Steenberghe D. Treatment of fenestration and dehiscence bone defects around oral implants using the guided tissue regeneration technique: a prospective multicenter study. Int J Oral Maxillofac Implants. **1995** May – Jun; 10(3): 312 – 318.

Dahlin C, Lekholm U, Becker W, Becker B, Higuchi K, Callens A, van Steenberghe D. Treatment of fenestration and dehiscence bone defects around oral implants using the guided tissue regeneration technique: a prospective multicenter study. Int J Oral Maxillofac Implants. **1995** May – Jun; 10(3): 312 – 318.

Dahlin C, Simion M, Hatano N. Long-term follow-up on soft and hard tissue levels following guided bone regeneration treatment in combination with a xenogeneic filling material: a 5-year prospective clinical study. Clin Implant Dent Relat Res. **2010** Dec; 12(4): 263 – 270.

De Boever AL, De Boever JA. Guided bone regeneration around non-submerged implants in narrow alveolar ridges: a prospective long-term clinical study. Clin Oral Implants Res. **2005** Oct; 16(5): 549 – 556.

De Santis D, Trevisiol L, D'Agostino A, Cucchi A, De Gemmis A, Nocini PF. Guided bone regeneration with autogenous block grafts applied to Le Fort I osteotomy for treatment of severely resorbed maxillae: a 4- to 6-year prospective study. Clin Oral Implants Res. **2012** Jan; 23(1): 60 – 69.

Dietrich U, Lippold R, Dirmeier T, Beneke N, Wagner W. Statistische Ergebnisse zur Implantatprognose am Beispiel von 2017 IMZ-Implantaten unterschiedlicher Indikation der letzten 13 Jahre. Zeitschrift für zahnärztliche Implantologie. **1993**; 9: 9 – 18.

Donos N, Kostopoulos L, Karring T. Alveolar ridge augmentation using a resorbable copolymer membrane and autogenous bone grafts. An experimental study in the rat. Clin Oral Implants Res. **2002** Apr; 13(1): 203 – 213.

Donovan MG, Dickerson NC, Hanson LJ, Gustafson RB. Maxillary and mandibular reconstruction using calvarial bone grafts and Branemark implants: a preliminary report. J Oral Maxillofac Surg **1994** Jun; 52(6): 588 – 594.

Edwards SP. Computer-assisted craniomaxillofacial surgery. Oral Maxillofac Surg North Am. **2010** Feb; 22(1): 117 – 134.

Ellis E 3rd, McFadden D. The value of a diagnostic setup for full fixed maxillary implant prosthetics. J Oral Maxillofac Surg. **2007** Sep; 65(9): 1764–1771.

Engelstad ME, Morse T. Anterior iliac crest, posterior iliac crest, and proximal tibia donor sites: a comparison of cancellous bone volumes in fresh cadavers. J Oral Maxillofac Surg. **2010** Dec; 68(12): 3015–3021.

Esposito M, Grusovin MG, Patel S, Worthington HV, Coulthard P. Interventions for replacing missing teeth: hyperbaric oxygen therapy for irradiated patients who require dental implants. Cochrane Database Syst Rev. **2008** Jan 23; (1) CD003603.

Esposito M, Cannizzaro G, Bozzoli P, Checchi L, Ferri V, Landriani S, Leone M, Todisco M, Torchio C, Testori T, Galli F, Felice P. Effectiveness of prophylactic antibiotics at placement of dental implants: a pragmatic multicentre placebo-controlled randomised clinical trial. Eur J Oral Implantol. **2010** Summer; 3(2): 135–143.

Fugazzotto PA. Success and failure rates of osseointegrated implants in function in regenerated bone for 6 to 51 months: a preliminary report. Int J Oral Maxillofac Implants. **1997** Jan–Feb; 12(1): 17–24.

Gaggl A, Schultes G, Karcher H. Vertical alveolar ridge distraction with prosthetic treatable distractors: a clinical investigation. Int J Oral Maxillofac Implants. **2000** Sep–Oct; 15(5): 701–710.

Gallucci G, Bernard JP, Belser U. Immediate loading of eight implants in the maxilla and six implants in the mandible and final restoration with three-unit and four-unit FDPs. In: Wismeijer D, Casentini P, Gallucci G, Chiapasco M (eds). Loading protocols in implant dentistry – edentulous patients. ITI Treatment Guide, Vol 4. Berlin: Quintessence; **2010**: 177–186.

Geurs NC, Korostoff JM, Vassipulos PJ, Kang TH, Jeffcoat M, Kellar R, Reddy MS. Clinical and histological assessment of lateral alveolar ridge augmentation using a synthetic long-term bioresorbable membrane and an allograft. J Periodontol. **2008** Jul; 79(7): 1130–1140.

Gonzalez-Garcia R, Monje F, Moreno C. Alveolar split osteotomy for the treatment of the severe narrow ridge maxillary atrophy: a modified technique. Int J Oral Maxillofac Surg. **2011** Jan; 40(1): 57–64.

Gottlow J, Dard M, Kjellson F, Obrecht M, Sennerby L. Evaluation of a new titanium-zirconium dental implant: a biomechanical and histological comparative study in the mini pig. Clin Implant Dent Relat Res. **2012** Aug; 14(4): 538–545.

Grant BT, Amenedo C, Freeman K, Kraut RA. Outcomes of placing dental implants in patients taking oral bisphosphonates: A review of 115 cases. J Oral Maxillofac Surg. **2008** Feb; 66(2): 223–230.

Hämmerle CH, Lang NP. Single stage surgery combining transmucosal implant placement with guided bone regeneration and bioresorbable materials. Clin Oral Implants Res. **2001**; 12: 9–18.

Hämmerle CH, Jung RE, Yaman D, Lang NP. Ridge augmentation by applying bioresorbable membranes and deproteinized bovine bone mineral: a report of twelve consecutive cases. Clin Oral Implants Res. **2008** Jan; 19(1): 19–25.

Heitz-Mayfield LJ, Huynh-Ba G. History of treated periodontitis and smoking as risks for implant therapy. Int J Oral Maxillofac Implants. **2009**; 24 Suppl: 34–68.

Hürzeler MB, Kohal RJ, Naghshbandi J, Mota LF, Conradt J, Hutmacher D, Caffesse RG. Evaluation of a new bioresorbable barrier to facilitate guided bone regeneration around exposed implant threads. An experimental study in the monkey. Int J Oral Maxillofac Surg. **1998** Aug; 27(4): 315–320.

Isaksson S, Ekfeldt A, Alberius P, Blomqvist JE. Early results from reconstruction of severely atrophic (Class VI) maxillas by immediate endosseous implants in conjunction with bone grafting and Le Fort I osteotomy. Int J Oral Maxillofac Surg. **1993** Jun; 22(3): 144–148.

Jensen J, Sindet-Pedersen S. Autogenous mandibular bone grafts and osseointegrated implants for reconstruction of the severely atrophied maxilla: a preliminary report. J Oral Maxillofac Surg **1991** Dec; 49(12): 1277–1287.

Jensen OT, Cockrell R, Kuhlke L, Reed C. Anterior maxillary alveolar distraction osteogenesis: a prospective 5-year clinical study. Int J Oral Maxillofac Implants. **2002** Jan–Feb; 17(1): 52–68.

Jensen SS, Yeo A, Dard M, Hunziker E, Schenk R, Buser D. Evaluation of a novel biphasic calcium phosphate in standardized bone defects: a histologic and histomorphometric study in the mandibles of minipigs. Clin Oral Implants Res. **2007** Dec; 18(6): 752–760.

Jensen SS, Terheyden H. Bone augmentation procedures in localized defects in the alveolar ridge: clinical results with different bone grafts and bone-substitute materials. Int J Oral Maxillofac Implants. **2009**; 24 Suppl: 218–236.

Johnston BC, Ma SS, Goldenberg JZ, Thorlund K, Vandvik PO, Loeb M, Guyatt GH. Probiotics for the prevention of Clostridium difficile-associated diarrhea: a systematic review and meta-analysis. Ann Intern Med. **2012** Dec; 157(12): 878–888.

Jung R, Haig GA, Thoma DS, Hämmerle CH. A randomized, controlled clinical trial to evaluate a new membrane for guided bone regeneration around dental implants. Clin Oral Implants Res. **2009** Feb; 20(2): 162–168.

Kahnberg KE, Nilsson P, Rasmusson L. Le Fort I osteotomy with interpositional bone grafts and implants for rehabilitation of the severely resorbed maxilla: a 2-stage procedure. Int J Oral Maxillofac Implants. **1999** Jul–Aug; 14(4): 571–578.

Karageorgiou V, Kaplan D. Porosity of 3D biomaterial scaffolds and osteogenesis. Biomaterials. **2005** Sep; 26(27): 5474–5491.

Katsuyama H, Jensen SS. Treatment options for sinus floor elevation. In: Chen S, Buser D, Wismeijer D (eds): Sinus floor elevation procedures. ITI Treatment Guide, Vol 5. Berlin: Quintessence; **2011**: 33–57.

Kleinheinz J, Büchter A, Kruse-Lösler B, Weingart D, Joos U. Incision design in implant dentistry based on vascularization of the mucosa. Clin Oral Impl Res. **2005** Oct; 16(5): 518–523.

Kobayashi E, Matsumoto S, Doi H, Yoneyama T, Hamanaka H. Mechanical properties of the binary titanium-zirconium alloys and their potential for biomedical materials. J Biomed Mater Res. **1995** Aug; 29(8): 943–950.

Kumar MN, Honne T. Survival of dental implants in bisphosphonate users versus non-users: a systematic review. Eur J Prosthodont Restor Dent. **2012** Dec; 20(4): 159–162.

Langer B. Spontaneous in situ gingival augmentation. Int J Periodontics Restorative Dent. **1994** Dec; 14(6): 524–535.

Li KK, Stephens WL, Gliklich R. Reconstruction of the severely atrophic edentulous maxilla using Le Fort I osteotomy with simultaneous bone graft and implant placement. J Oral Maxillofac Surg. **1996** May; 54(5): 542–546.

Llambes F, Silvestre FJ, Caffesse R. Vertical guided bone regeneration with bioabsorbable barriers. J Periodontol. **2007** Oct; 78(10): 2036–2042.

Lorenzoni M, Pertl C, Polansky R, Wegscheider W. Guided bone regeneration with barrier membranes—a clinical and radiographic follow-up study after 24 months. Clin Oral Implants Res. **1999** Feb; 10(1): 16–23.

Lundgren S, Nyström E, Nilson H, Gunne J, Lindhagen O. Bone grafting to the maxillary sinuses, nasal floor and anterior maxilla in the atrophic edentulous maxilla. Int J Oral Maxillofac Surg. **1997** Dec; 26(6): 428–434.

Lundgren S, Sennerby L. Bone Reformation. Contemporary bone augmentation procedures in oral and maxillofacial implant surgery. Berlin: Quintessenz; **2008**.

Lundgren S, Sjöström M, Nyström E, Sennerby L. Strategies in reconstruction of the atrophic maxilla with autogenous bone grafts and endosseous implants. Periodontol 2000; **2008**; 47: 143–161.

Maiorana C, Beretta M, Salina S, Santoro F. Reduction of autogenous bone graft resorption by means of Bio-Oss coverage: a prospective study. Int J Periodontics Restorative Dent. **2005** Feb; 25(1): 19–25.

Marchetti C, Corinaldesi G, Pieri F, Degidi M, Piattelli A. Alveolar distraction osteogenesis for bone augmentation of severely atrophic ridges in 10 consecutive cases: a histologic and histomorphometric study. J Periodontol. **2007** Feb; 78(2): 360–366.

Mardas N, Kostopoulos L, Stavropoulos A, Karring T. Evaluation of a cell-permeable barrier for guided tissue regeneration combined with demineralized bone matrix. Clin Oral Implants Res. **2003** Dec; 14(6): 812–828.

Martin WC, Morton D, Buser D. Pre-operative analysis and prosthetic treatment planning in esthetic implant dentistry. In: Buser D, Belser UC, Wismeijer D (eds): ITI Treatment Guide, Vol 1: Single tooth replacement in the anterior maxilla. Berlin: Quintessenz; **2006**: 9–24.

Marx RE. Pamidronate (Aredia) and zoledronate (Zometa) induced avascular necrosis of the jaws: A growing epidemic. J Oral Maxillofacial Surg. **2003** Sep; 61(9): 1115–1118.

McGrath CJ, Schepers SH, Blijdorp PA, Hoppenreijs TJ, Erbe M. Simultaneous placement of endosteal implants and mandibular onlay grafting for treatment of the atrophic mandible. A preliminary report. Int J Oral Maxillofac Surg. **1996** Jun; 25(3): 184–188.

Meijndert L, Raghoebar GM, Schupbach P, Meijer HJ, Vissink A. Bone quality at the implant site after reconstruction of a local defect of the maxillary anterior ridge with chin bone or deproteinised cancellous bovine bone. Int J Oral Maxillofac Surg. **2005** Dec; 34(8): 877–884.

Merli M, Migani M, Esposito M. Vertical ridge augmentation with autogenous bone grafts: resorbable barriers supported by osteosynthesis plates versus titanium-reinforced barriers. A preliminary report of a blinded, randomized controlled clinical trial. Int J Oral Maxillofac Implants. **2007** May–Jun; 22(3): 373–382.

Milinkovic I, Cordaro L. Are there specific indications for the different bone augmentation procedures? A systematic review. Int J Oral Maxillofac Surg. **2013** (submitted for publication).

Miron RJ, Hedbom E, Saulacic N, Zhang Y, Sculean A, Bosshardt DD, Buser D. Osteogenic potential of autogenous bone grafts harvested with four different surgical techniques. J Dent Res. **2011** Dec; 90(2): 1428–1433.

Misch CE. Bone classification, training keys to implant success. Dent Today. **1989** May; 8(4): 39–44.

Nemcovsky CE, Artzi Z, Moses O, Gelernter I. Healing of dehiscence defects at delayed-immediate implant sites primarily closed by a rotated palatal flap following extraction. Int J Oral Maxillofac Implants. **2000** Jul–Aug; 15(4): 550–558.

Neyt LF, De Clercq CA, Abeloos JV, Mommaerts MY. Reconstruction of the severely resorbed maxilla with a combination of sinus augmentation, onlay bone grafting, and implants. J Oral Maxillofac Surg. **1997** Dec; 55(12): 1397–1401.

Nissan J, Ghelfan O, Mardinger O, Calderon S, Chaushu G. Efficacy of cancellous block allograft augmentation prior to implant placement in the posterior atrophic mandible. Clin Implant Dent Relat Res. **2011** Dec; 13(4): 279–285.

Nkenke E, Schultze-Mosgau S, Radespiel-Tröger M, Kloss F, Neukam FW. Morbidity of harvesting of chin grafts: A prospective study. Clin Oral Implants Res. **2001**; 12: 495–502.

Nyman S, Lang NP, Buser D, Brägger U. Bone regeneration adjacent to titanium dental implants using guided tissue regeneration: a report of two cases. Int J Oral Maxillofac Implants. **1990** Spring; 5(1): 9–14.

Nyman, SR, Lang NP. Guided tissue regeneration and dental implants. Periodontology 2000. **1994**; 4: 109–118.

Nyström E, Nilson H, Gunne J, Lundgren S. Reconstruction of the atrophic maxilla with interpositional bone grafting/Le Fort I osteotomy and endosteal implants: an 11–16 year follow-up. Int J Oral Maxillofac Surg. **2009** Jan; 38(1): 1–6.

Oates TW. Bisphosphonates: a hindrance or a help? Int J Oral Maxillofac Implants, **2013** May–Jun; 28(3): 655–657.

Park SH, Lee KW, Oh TJ, Misch CE, Shotwell J, Wang HL. Effect of absorbable membranes on sandwich bone augmentation. Clin Oral Implants Res. **2008** Jan; 19(1): 32–41.

Parodi R, Carusi G, Santarelli G, Nanni F. Implant placement in large edentulous ridges expanded by GBR using a bioresorbable collagen membrane. Int J Periodontics Restorative Dent. **1998** Jun; 18(3): 266–275.

Peleg M, Chaushu G, Blinder D, Taicher S. Use of lyodura for bone augmentation of osseous defects around dental implants. J Periodontol. **1999** Aug; 70(8): 853–860.

Proussaefs P, Lozada J. The use of intraorally harvested autogenous block grafts for vertical alveolar ridge augmentation: A human study. Int J Periodontics Restorative Dent. **2005**; 25: 351–363.

Rachmiel A, Srouji S, Peled M. Alveolar ridge augmentation by distraction osteogenesis. Int J Oral Maxillofac Surg. **2001** Dec; 30(6): 510–517.

Raghoebar GM, Louwerse C, Kalk WW, Vissink A. Morbidity of chin bone harvesting. Clin Oral Implants Res. **2001**; 12: 503–507.

Ramel CF, Wismeijer DA, Hämmerle CH, Jung RE: A randomized, controlled clinical evaluation of a synthetic gel membrane for guided bone regeneration around dental implants: clinical and radiologic 1- and 3-year results. Int J Oral Maxillofac Implants. **2012** Mar–Apr; 27(2): 435–441.

Reissmann DR, Dietze B, Vogeler M, Schmelzeisen R, Heydecke G. Impact of donor site for bone graft harvesting for dental implants on health-related and oral health-related quality of life. Clin Oral Implants Res. **2013** Jun; 24(6): 698 – 705.

Robiony M, Zorzan E, Polini F, Sembronio S, Toro C, Politi M. Osteogenesis distraction and platelet-rich plasma: combined use in restoration of severe atrophic mandible. Long-term results. Clin Oral Implants Res. **2008** Nov; 19(11): 1202 – 1210.

Rocchietta I. Fontana F. Simion, M. Clinical outcomes of vertical bone augmentation to enable dental implant placement: a systematic review. J Clin Periodontol. **2008**; 35: 203 – 215.

Roccuzzo M, Ramieri G, Bunino M, Berrone S. Autogenous bone graft alone or associated with titanium mesh for vertical alveolar ridge augmentation: a controlled clinical trial. Clin Oral Implants Res. **2007** Jun; 18(3): 286 – 294.

Roccuzzo M, Wilson TG Jr.: A prospective study of 3 weeks' loading of chemically modified titanium implants in the maxillary molar region: 1-year results; Int J Oral Maxillofac Implants. **2009** Jan – Feb; 24(1): 65 – 72.

Sanz I, Garcia-Gargallo M, Herrera D, Martin C, Figuero E, Sanz M. Surgical protocols for early implant placement in post-extraction sockets: a systematic review. Clin Oral Implants Res. **2012** Feb; 23 Suppl 5: 67 – 79.

Scheerlinck LM, Muradin MS, van der Bilt A, Meijer GJ, Koole R, Van Cann EM. Donor site complications in bone grafting: comparison of iliac crest, calvarial, and mandibular ramus bone; Int J Oral Maxillofac Implants. **2013** Jan – Feb; 28(1): 222 – 227.

Schenk RK, Buser D, Hardwick WR, Dahlin C. Healing pattern of bone regeneration in membrane-protected defects. A histologic study in the canine mandible. Int J Oral Maxillofac Implants. **1994** Jan; 9(1): 13 – 29.

Schettler D. Sandwich-Technik mit Knorpeltransplantat zur Alveolarkammerhöhung im Unterkiefer. [Sandwich technique with cartilage transplant for raising the alveolar process in the lower jaw]. Fortschr Kiefer Gesichtschir. **1976**; 20: 61 – 63.

Schratt HE, Regel G, Kiesewetter B, Tscherne H. HIV-Infektion durch kältekonservierte Knochentransplantate. [HIV infection caused by cold preserved bone transplants.] Unfallchirurg. **1996** Sep; 99(9): 679 – 684.

Schwartz-Arad D, Levin L. Intraoral autogenous block onlay bone grafting for extensive reconstruction of atrophic maxillary alveolar ridges. J Periodontol. **2005** Apr; 76(4): 636 – 641.

Sethi A, Kaus T. Maxillary ridge expansion with simultaneous implant placement: 5-year results of an ongoing clinical study. Int J Oral Maxillofac Implants. **2000** Jul – Aug; 15(4): 491 – 499.

Sethi A, Kaus T. Ridge augmentation using mandibular block bone grafts: Preliminary results of an ongoing prospective study. Int J Oral Maxillofac Implants. **2001** May – Jun; 16(3): 378 – 388.

Simion M, Jovanovic SA, Tinti C, Benfenati SP. Long-term evaluation of osseointegrated implants inserted at the time or after vertical ridge augmentation. A retrospective study on 123 implants with 1 – 5 years follow-up. Clin Oral Implants Res. **2001** Feb; 12(1): 35 – 45.

Simion M, Fontana F, Rasperini G, Maiorana C. Vertical ridge augmentation by expanded-polytetrafluoro-ethylene membrane and a combination of intraoral autogenous bone graft and deproteinized anorganic bovine bone (Bio Oss). Clin Oral Implants Res. **2007** Oct; 18(5): 620 – 629.

Simonds RJ. HIV transmission by organ and tissue transplantation. AIDS. **1993** Nov; 7 Suppl 2: S35 – 38.

Simonpieri A, Del Corso M, Sammartino G, Dohan Ehrenfest DM. The relevance of Choukroun's platelet-rich fibrin and metronidazole during complex maxillary rehabilitations using bone allograft. Part I: a new grafting protocol. Implant Dent. **2009** Apr; 18(2): 102 – 111.

Smolka W, Bosshardt DD, Mericske-Stern R, Iizuka T. Reconstruction of the severely atrophic mandible using calvarial split bone grafts for implant-supported oral rehabilitation. Oral Surg Oral Med Oral Pathol Oral Radiol Endod. **2006** Jan; 101(1): 35 – 42.

Sohn DS, Lee HJ, Heo JU, Moon JW, Park IS, Romanos GE. Immediate and delayed lateral ridge expansion technique in the atrophic posterior mandibular ridge. J Oral Maxillofac Surg. **2010** Sep; 68(9): 2283 – 2290.

Springer IN, Terheyden H, Geiss S, Härle F, Hedderich J, Açil Y. Particulated bone grafts—effectiveness of bone cell supply. Clin Oral Implants Res. **2004** Apr; 15(2): 205-212.

Steiner M, Ramp WK. Endosseous dental implants and the glucocorticoid-dependent patient. J Oral Implantol. **1990**; 16(3): 211–217.

Stellingsma K, Slagter AP, Stegenga B, Raghoebar GM, Meijer HJ. Masticatory function in patients with an extremely resorbed mandible restored with mandibular implant-retained overdentures: comparison of three types of treatment protocols. J Oral Rehabil. **2005** Jun; 32(6): 403–410.

Stewart RE, Witkop Jr CJ, Bixler D. The dentition and anomalies of tooth size, form, structure, and eruption. In: Stewart RE, Barber TK, Troutman KC, Wei SHY, eds. Pediatric Dentistry: Scientific Foundations of Clinical Procedures. 1st ed. St. Louis: CV Mosby; **1982**: 87–109.

Stoelinga PJ, Slagter AP, Brouns JJ. Rehabilitation of patients with severe (Class VI) maxillary resorption using Le Fort I osteotomy, interposed bone grafts and endosteal implants: 1–8 years follow-up on a two-stage procedure. Int J Oral Maxillofac Surg. **2000** Jun; 29(3): 188–193.

Sun HL, Huang C, Wu YR, Shi B. Failure rates of short (≤ 10 mm) dental implants and factors influencing their failure: a systematic review. Int J Oral Maxillofac Implants. **2011** Jul–Aug; 26(4): 816–825.

Tan WC, Ong M, Han J, Mattheos N, Pjetursson BE, Tsai AY, Sanz I, Wong MC, Lang NP; on behalf of the ITI Antibiotic Study Group. Effect of systemic antibiotics on clinical and patient-reported outcomes of implant therapy—a multicenter randomized controlled clinical trial. Clin Oral Implants Res. **2013** Jan 24. [Epub ahead of print]

Telleman G, Raghoebar GM, Vissink A, den Hartog L, Huddleston Slater JJ, Meijer HJ. A systematic review of the prognosis of short (<10 mm) dental implants placed in the partially edentulous patient. J Clin Periodontol. **2011** Jul; 38(7): 667–676.

Terheyden H. Knochenaugmentationen in der Implantologie. [Bone augmentation in implantology.] Dtsch Zahnärztl Z **2010**; 65: 320–331.

Todisco M. Early loading of implants in vertically augmented bone with non-resorbable membranes and deproteinised anorganic bovine bone. An uncontrolled prospective cohort study. Eur J Oral Implantol. **2010** Spring; 3(1): 47–58.

Triplett RG, Schow SR. Autologous bone grafts and endosseous implants: complementary techniques. J Oral Maxillofac Surg. **1996** Apr; 54(4): 486–494.

Urist MR. Bone: formation by autoinduction. Science **1965**; 150: 893–899.

van Steenberghe D, Callens A, Geers L, Jacobs R. The clinical use of deproteinized bovine bone mineral on bone regeneration in conjunction with immediate implant installation. Clin Oral Implants Res. **2000** Jun; 11(3): 210–216

Vignoletti F, Matesanz P, Rodrigo D, Figuero E, Martin C, Sanz M. Surgical protocols for ridge preservation after tooth extraction. A systematic review. Clin Oral Implants Res. **2012** Feb; 23 Suppl 5: 22–38.

von Arx T, Wallkamm B, Hardt N. Localized ridge augmentation using a micro titanium mesh: a report on 27 implants followed from 1 to 3 years after functional loading. Clin Oral Implants Res. **1998** Apr; 9(2): 123–130.

von Arx T, Cochran DL, Hermann J, Schenk RK, Higginbottom F, Buser D. Lateral ridge augmentation and implant placement: an experimental study evaluating implant osseointegration in different augmentation materials in the canine mandible. Int J Oral Maxillofac Implants. **2001** May–Jun; 16(3): 343–354.

von Arx T, Hafliger J, Chappuis V. Neurosensory disturbances following bone harvesting in the symphysis: a prospective clinical study. Clin Oral Implants Res. **2005** Aug; 16(4): 432–439.

von Arx T, Buser D. Horizontal ridge augmentation using autogenous block grafts and the guided bone regeneration technique with collagen membranes: A clinical study with 42 patients. Clin Oral Implants Res. **2006** Aug; 17(4): 359–366.

von Arx T, Buser D. Guided bone regeneration and autogenous block grafts for horizontal ridge augmentation: a staged approach. In: Buser D (ed): 20 years of guided bone regeneration in implant dentistry. 2nd ed. Chicago: Quintessence; **2009**, 195–229.

Wallace S, Gellin R. Clinical evaluation of freeze-dried cancellous block allografts for ridge augmentation and implant placement in the maxilla. Implant Dent. **2010** Aug; 19(4): 272–279.

Wang HL, Weber D, McCauley LK. Effect of long-term oral bisphosphonates on implant wound healing: literature review and a case report. J Periodontol. **2007** Mar; 78(3): 584–594.

Weingart D, ten Bruggenkate CM. (2000), Treatment of fully edentulous patients with ITI implants . Clinical Oral Implants Research. **2000**; 11 Suppl 1: 69–82.

Widmark G, Ivanoff CJ. Augmentation of exposed implant threads with autogenous bone chips: prospective clinical study. Clin Implant Dent Relat Res. **2000**; 2(4): 178–183.

Wiltfang J, Jätschmann N, Hedderich J, Neukam FW, Schlegel KA, Gierloff M. Effect of deproteinized bovine bone matrix coverage on the resorption of iliac cortico-spongeous bone grafts—a prospective study of two cohorts. Clin Oral Implants Res. **2012** Nov 27. doi: 10.1111/clr.12074. [Epub ahead of print]

Yildirim M, Hanisch O, Spiekermann H. Simultaneous hard and soft tissue augmentation for implant-supported single-tooth restorations. Pract Periodontics Aesthet Dent. **1997** Nov–Dec; 9(9): 1023–1031.

Zitzmann NU, Naef R, Schärer P. Resorbable versus non-resorbable membranes in combination with Bio-Oss for guided bone regeneration. Int J Oral Maxillofac Implants. **1997** Nov–Dec; 12(6): 844–852.